# bumpin'

# THE MODERN GUIDE TO PREGNANCY

### NAVIGATING THE WILD, WEIRD, AND WONDERFUL JOURNEY
### FROM CONCEPTION THROUGH BIRTH AND BEYOND

# bumpin'

## leslie schrock

Tiller Press

New York   London   Toronto   Sydney   New Delhi

TILLER PRESS

Tiller Press
An Imprint of Simon & Schuster, Inc.
1230 Avenue of the Americas
New York, NY 10020

First Tiller Press trade paperback edition December 2019

TILLER PRESS and colophon are trademarks of Simon & Schuster, Inc.

This publication contains the opinions and ideas of its author. It is intended to provide helpful and informative material on the subjects addressed in the publication. It is sold with the understanding that the author and publisher are not engaged in rendering medical, health, or any other kind of personal professional services in the book. The reader should consult his or her medical, health or other competent professional before adopting any of the suggestions in this book or drawing inferences from it. The author and publisher specifically disclaim all responsibility for any liability, loss or risk, personal or otherwise, which is incurred as a consequence, directly or indirectly, of the use and application of any of the contents of this book.

For information about special discounts for bulk purchases, please contact Simon & Schuster Special Sales at 1-866-506-1949 or business@simonandschuster.com.

The Simon & Schuster Speakers Bureau can bring authors to your live event. For more information or to book an event, contact the Simon & Schuster Speakers Bureau at 1-866-248-3049 or visit our website at www.simonspeakers.com.

Interior design by Jennifer Chung

Manufactured in the United States of America

3   5   7   9   10   8   6   4   2

Library of Congress Control Number: 2019947486

ISBN 978-1-9821-3044-2
ISBN 978-1-9821-3045-9 (ebook)

*To Mr. Baby—you were worth the wait*
*And to Nick, who was by my side through it all*

It's no use going back to yesterday,
because I was a different person then.

—Lewis Carroll, *Alice's Adventures in Wonderland*

# CONTENTS

# FOREWORD

Obstetrics is daunting. Unlike other medical specialties, there are two patients—two hearts asynchronously beating and two sets of expectations, both fragile and intertwined. Not to mention familial and cultural inheritances that often go well beyond those two lives. The practice of obstetrics has evolved more slowly than other fields, for various reasons: the challenges of performing randomized controlled trials on a mother-fetal cohort; the dramatic physiological changes that happen during pregnancy; ethical considerations around safety; fear of the maternal body; and a light sprinkling of misogyny to boot.

Personally, I pursued a career in obstetrics-gynecology because I was fascinated by gynecologic surgery. In a peripatetic turn, I now spend my professional life thinking about how we can improve safety as we deliver complex coordinated care to mothers in Labor and Delivery. As an OB hospitalist, I witness the fruition of months of careful planning, and have come to understand some of the common frustrations and elations of birthing women.

My other job is as medical director for Maven Clinic, a telehealth platform for women and families. I help design and implement care for women across twenty women's health specialties and among sixteen hundred practitioners. In both of these positions, safety, outcomes data, and a multidisciplinary team are essential. As you may know, there are many maternal and neonatal indices which need improvement. Women—and children—deserve not only better care, but to have gaps in their care closed. Our work is difficult but necessary. And the more good information patients have about their own bodies, the better the outcomes are.

As a practicing ob-gyn, I cannot divorce my mind from the pedagogy of medicine—the manner in which physicians are inculcated, the analysis we perform when confronted with clinical conditions, the hierarchy of our training and practice. But obstetrics is so much more than facts in a medical school textbook. The wisdom that many doctors bring to obstetrics comes from a range of sources: midwives who have shared expertise on maternal positions in labor; maternal-fetal medicine specialists who contextualized complex genetic abnormalities; doulas who demonstrate how to center the pregnant woman in her particular narrative; labor nurses whose wisdom, laughter, advocacy, and sheer tenacity keep us sane day after day. And let's be honest, our own experience—carrying my twins and becoming a mother certainly taught me a thing or two as well. Obstetrics is a team sport.

In medicine, we contend with physiological limits: blood pressure and heart rates, hormones and neurotransmitters. With the architecture of birth: the bones of the maternal pelvis can expand only so much. With physics: a uterus has only so much power to push the infant out against opposing forces. And with the senses: a maternal body can withstand only a finite amount of pain. With all the technology available to us, we sometimes forget that the process of pregnancy and birth is a mixture of physiology, environment, mostly genetics, and a bit of unexplained randomness. We can treat things like preterm labor and preeclampsia when they occur, but we are less adept at predicting to whom those things will happen, and instead rely on risk factors and demographics. I am consistently surprised that healthy women can sometimes have the most complicated pregnancies, and women with serious risk factors can avoid any complications at all. And of course, I understand that for women, the process of pregnancy and birth—unlike almost any other medical condition—isn't about simply avoiding risk. It's about creating a family. Ideally, there is room for both languages to be spoken and heard.

From the patient's perspective, the practice of obstetrics may not feel as collaborative as we would like, in part because we don't always do the best job of talking across our respective aisles, but also because there are thousands of information sources for women to turn to today. What I haven't seen among these sources is a book that combines the rigor and precision of the best medical literature with the wisdom of specialists from a variety of disciplines, training, and backgrounds— and delivers it with the expert reassurance of personal experience. Leslie Schrock, in this book, has done just that not only for the process of pregnancy itself, but fertility, conception, and all things postpartum. Though the task of apprehending good science from pseudoscience is daunting, especially given the overwhelming amount of information online, Leslie understands that we owe it to women and families to try.

As I assisted in the medical editing of this book, I looked to add sources based on the latest research available, knowing that science is iterative, and what holds true today may change in years to come. Having been chair of an OB-GYN department, I'm aware that old practices sometimes take too long to die out. I have found that physicians, especially while committed to the scientific method, often bristle at changing their practice. Metrics, protocols, and outcomes data help, but so does humor, humility, and grace.

I hope you find answers to most of your questions in these pages, and perhaps even seek out the primary sources listed here. I also hope you feel embraced by these pages, and by Leslie's effervescent, uncensored warmth. Most of all, I hope this book makes accessible the insider information and medical truths that should guide your own decisions. Every pregnant woman deserves that.

Pregnancy and childbirth can bring us indescribable joy—and sometimes extreme pain. The process of making new life is unavoidably messy and raw, but ideally we emerge transformed, in the best sense. There's no right way to have a child; it has always been a collaboration between patient, practitioner, family, and friends. I've been privileged to share in so many of those journeys, and I can say with great confidence that you're lucky to have Leslie Schrock along on yours.

Jane van Dis, MD, FACOG

# PREFACE

I was pregnant for almost sixteen consecutive months before I had my son. The same time it takes to gestate a baby rhinoceros.

The first pregnancy ended early. I miscarried while traveling in British Columbia.

The second started just two weeks later. It was declared not viable at twelve weeks.

The third pregnancy began after a two-month break. My son, the baby rhino, was pulled out of my belly wailing nine months later.

Those sixteen months taught me a lot.

I learned that it's possible to get pregnant every cycle you try, even if you are *shudder* over thirty-five. That your body can take repeated hormonal punishment and stretching in strange places and still be strong. That giving up wine is a small sacrifice in the scheme of things. That even with optimism and preparation, birth, breastfeeding, and so many parts of the journey will not go as you plan. That knowledge, honesty, a sense of humor, and great friendships are the best weapons if you want to get through it intact. And that there is so much about pregnancy that no one talks about.

The last point especially came as a bit of a shock. After a decade in San Francisco's health tech scene, I've seen—and tried—a lot. From having my microbiome sequenced and getting my telomeres measured, to helping launch companies and giving talks around the world, I came into the experience with a lot more knowledge than most. So it was surprising to realize that even with my background, when it came to pregnancy I was totally clueless. And if the whole thing was a big box of ¯\\_(ツ)_/¯ to me, what was it like for everyone else?

So I bought or borrowed every book I could find, scanned academic journals for new research, learned how obstetricians are trained, and applied all of this knowledge to my adventure and, later, this book. Deciding to turn my little excavation into a book was almost as surprising as the varying opinions and conflicting research it unearthed.

On one side of the resource spectrum I found dense, clinical walls of text that covered every single possible health condition and were so dry they put me to sleep. They increased my paranoia about even the smallest twinges and led to many frantic googling sessions.

On the other end were the unsubstantiated opinions by self-styled "experts," devoid of facts and presented in language so patronizing one would assume the intended audience was the baby. I did not identify with the incessant *mama*-ing and felt that I would be judged for any deviations from "natural" frameworks.

By the end, all I could wonder is why a middle ground was so hard to find when ultimately everyone wants the same thing—healthy moms and babies.

There were also topics that neither side touched. For example, after jumping down the rabbit hole of fertility issues, I learned that after two years of trying, 10 percent of all couples still can't conceive,[1] and miscarriages happen in as many as one in three pregnancies.[2] As common as miscarriage is, if it was addressed at all, it was hidden at the very end of the book.

The history of childbirth also proved to be revealing. While modern medicine is responsible for incredible reductions in maternal and infant mortality rates, the emotional support that used to be a basic standard of care—before, during, and after delivery—has all but disappeared. This is changing with the resurgence of midwives and the growing use of doulas, but still has a long way to go.

One of the most mysterious areas I explored was the seldom-discussed fourth trimester and all its emotional and physical complexities. Knowing postpartum depression affects as many as one in five women,[3] the silence around its existence and root causes was, frankly, confusing. But if you combine the "snap-back" photos influencers post of their post-baby bodies (without the context of the time, effort, and re-sources required to achieve them), the lack of breastfeeding resources at work, and the general dearth of support for parents with all the tension of being a mother, someone's partner, and a professional, it starts to make sense. Add that public mommy shaming for doing the slightest thing "wrong" is carried out by the last people you'd expect—other mothers—and you have an environment primed for anxiety, stress, and yes, depression.

While we have a long way to go in supporting families, the care we provide to pregnant women is evolving, in part because technology enables more on-demand, affordable guidance than ever before. Advanced testing provides more insight into your fertility, and your developing baby. And with the many ovulation-tracking apps and tele-medicine options and sensors, it's never been easier to get answers when and where you need them. However, beware as message boards and social media are also full of advice that contradicts medical knowledge. And since Dr. Google is available anytime, he's often the first source we check.

One of the most popular pregnancy tomes was written in 1984 when first-time mothers were, on average, twenty-three years old.[4] Today the average age is closer to twenty-seven,[5] and as high as thirty-three in cities like San Francisco and New York.[6] Egg freezing, IVF, and more advanced early testing have extended childbearing years into the forties. Even with updates, most resources just aren't written with today's women in mind.

After an introduction to different practitioners during my years as an adviser to Maven, the family benefits platform, I grew my own care team and tried as many modalities as I could as research for this book. Acupuncture helped with first-trimester blahs, a physical therapist worked out aches and pains, a doula team explained what really happens during birth, pelvic floor physical therapy meant I avoided diastasis recti, all in combination with prenatal care by my crack team of ob-gyns.

This huge period of forced personal growth turned out to be great preparation for becoming a parent. Because try as I might, even with experts to lean on and all of this knowledge, I had to accept that I had little control over what happened. A good thing, too, because nothing really went the way we planned.

## THIS BOOK'S PERSPECTIVE

On that note, my explicit goal is *not* to focus on things that are frequently out of your control, or to perpetuate the idea that all pregnancies are exactly the same. So if you are looking for a second-by-second daily breakdown of your changing body or growing baby, this is probably not the book for you.

Instead, read on for a mix of science, practical advice, and a dash of personal experience—the information you need without all the detail you really don't. Written in real-time during my pregnancy and after my son arrived, it combines the latest clinical research with practical advice on topics like financial planning, what to buy, and how to handle your changing relationship. And it doesn't skip the hard parts, like fertility issues, miscarriage, and the postpartum period. Or real talk about topics like CBD. And the questions you may be too embarrassed to ask, like, will sleeping on my stomach hurt the baby? (Nope!)

Pregnancy is presented here as five trimesters versus the traditional three. Trimester zero is conception, one through three are the weeks baking your wee human, and four is the first three months postpartum. Each trimester starts with symptoms and solutions, advice for your partner, and a to-do list. The individual sections in each trimester go deeper to tackle the major decisions and events you'll face at each stage.

Another goal of this book is to remove the judgment around "natural" pregnancy and childbirth. Yes, our bodies are biologically designed to give birth. Humans have done it billions of times. However, utilizing assistance by choice or necessity, or encountering difficulty during birth, breastfeeding, or at any other time does not make you a failure, nor does it marginalize your experience. For that reason, pain medications and interventions during birth will be referred to as medicated or unmedicated, and birth types as vaginal or C-section.

Personalized medicine, or the idea that not all health treatments should be one-size-fits-all, is another concept that may be new. Every single pregnancy and baby is different, and just because something worked for your friend or sister doesn't mean it will for you. Happily, there are more tools than ever to individualize your care. Sections that cover finding the right providers, evaluating prenatal testing, and debunking long-held myths in areas like exercise and food are written in that spirit.

If you're picking up this book because you want to understand what your partner or friend or surrogate is experiencing, good for you! Flip to the beginning of each trimester for ways to be helpful and tangible things to do and to learn about the big changes in store.

I am not a medical professional. I am a curious person who felt disappointed by the lack of trustworthy resources available to women to make decisions during pregnancy, and as a result, the lack of confidence we sometimes feel as we go through it. For that reason, health guidelines were edited by an equally curious ob-gyn with many years of experience and training. Also tapped were nurse practitioners, therapists, midwives, doulas, ob-gyns, pelvic floor experts, trainers, physical therapists, and acupuncturists.

## THE DATA

Now let's get to the serious stuff. There is understandable ethical concern about exposing pregnant women and babies to the risks of research, hence why many studies are done with animals, have low sample sizes, or rely on self-reported data. New findings can change the minds of even the most august medical organizations, and widely circulated studies are sometimes later proven incorrect.

Clinical medicine is an average of seventeen years behind research,[7] and even the time required to categorize a drug's full risk profile is a whopping twenty-seven years after release.[8] So even with the urgency to probe maternal health's unexplored corners, research is slow to move from labs and papers into patient care.

Inherent bias, or known leanings that influence decision-making, is another issue. Whether it takes the form of confirmation bias (seeking evidence that confirms our first or existing impression), excessive coherence (using sparse evidence to quickly form coherent narratives, ignoring contradictions or nuance), or availability bias (overvaluing the most recent evidence), this, too, can impact findings and the frameworks for studies. Also at play is who or what organization is actually funding the research.

Disclaimers and wishes for more definitive answers aside, all studies are cited, and effort has been made to use the most well-vetted, current information available. The clinical practices come from trusted medical organizations, and are the same as the guidance you'll hear from your own ob-gyn or midwife.

## A FINAL NOTE BEFORE YOU START

Starting a family is rarely a straightforward journey. And even if things are smooth, it's a long one, as the average pregnancy is 280 days, or 6,720 hours long. This is the first of many reminders that asking for help doesn't make you weak or incompetent. Childbearing and child-rearing has always taken a village, and there is no better time to prepare for that reality than before your tiny human shows up.

I hope this book leaves you empowered to face whatever this wild, weird, and wonderful journey throws your way, teaches you at least one fact worth repeating, and is as fun for you to read as it was for me to write.

*Note: For those starting this journey as part of the LGBTQ or nonbinary communities, we standardize the pronouns* she *and* her, *and refer to the birth parent as a woman and mother for purposes of simplicity to all readers.*

# Trimester Zero

**W**elcome to the wild, sometimes painful, emotional, magical journey that is becoming a parent. Whether you are just starting, accompanying someone else, or pondering it in the future, deciding to conceive is the first of many life-changing moments to come.

Conception, and later pregnancy and birth, often feels like it's happening *to* you versus following a script of what it *should* be like. Here is another reminder that there are no shoulds in this process, and that unfortunately you are not in full control even if you do everything "right." The journey will be unique to you, just like your eventual baby. So try not to compare your experience to those of friends and family, or to stories you read online.

Nature's independent agenda aside, there are some choices you can control, and conception is your first opportunity to optimize your care, body, and life. Trimester Zero covers how to get your bodies (that's right—yours and your partner's) and lives ready. Next comes a refresher on how making a baby really works. This is useful if your only formal training was during middle school sex ed, as technology and our knowledge of the process have improved in the years since.

The lack of transparency and mythology around complications will never change unless we talk about them. So whether it's for you or someone you love, read about the challenges (without letting them freak you out), find out what to do if you run into them, and discover the wide range of solutions that exist to build a family today.

*Greetings, friend! To separate the facts from the personal commentary, these italicized sections appear as notes throughout to recount my somewhat challenging journey through this process. If you're just here for the science, feel free to skip 'em. But if you do decide to read on, I promise to be brutally honest and try not to leave anything out.*

## FOR PARTNERS

Welcome to team conception, partners. Though your role (and you) will often be secondary, there are plenty of ways to feel involved throughout the pregnancy and after birth. These sections are designed to help you sidestep common issues couples encounter at each phase, navigate the ways your lives will change, and provide suggestions to keep your relationship healthy.

### *Take your lifestyle and health seriously*

Society's focus before, during, and even after pregnancy is mostly on the woman's contributions and choices. If conception is a struggle, the blame will fall squarely on her first—especially in regard to such indicators as egg quality and hormonal markers—not, if you are a heterosexual male, on you. Ironic, as at least 40 percent of fertility issues are related to sperm and men's health choices![1] So if things aren't happening, be proactive and offer to get yourself checked.

Even more important, start taking your own health more seriously. Given that you are (likely) providing half of your child's genetic material, what you do matters, too.

### *Be patient and keep things light*

Conception can quickly become a stressful and obsessive process, especially aspects like timing sex and calculating fertile windows. Add hormonal changes (if a woman just quit taking birth control) or worry when things don't happen immediately, and any joy in the creation of new life can vanish.

Your mission, should you choose to accept it: Be patient, and find ways to defuse the anxiety and keep things fun. Schedule a date night. Try to keep each other distracted, especially if getting pregnant takes a bit of time. Keep the lines of communication open. And even if you're not the type to talk about your feelings, be honest about how you are dealing, too.

# GET YOUR BODIES AND LIVES READY

### From genetic screenings to finances, sanity and a healthy pregnancy start before you conceive.

This section may feel like it's just for overachievers. Consider the below a menu of available options rather than a mandate. Conception, and later pregnancy and parenthood, is about stringing together the parts that feel right to you, and leaving those that don't.

Preparation for pregnancy is almost always focused on physical health—lifestyle cleanses, what to eat and do. While aspects like quitting birth control (and its accompanying gnarly hormone changes) are important to understand, if your partner is providing sperm, they should get to know how their lifestyle and health impact fertility and an eventual pregnancy. Their medical history, genetics, and daily choices are also major factors in conception.

It's not just about the raw materials. Most new parents will tell you their relationship changed after having a baby. Some shift in wonderful ways; for example, a couple may feel more bonded. Other changes are less appealing, like having limited time together and less frequent sex or intimacy, or experiencing feelings of bitterness tied

5

to lopsided responsibilities. And how could such a major event *not* change things?

Family therapists suggest talking about your individual and shared parenting and life expectations before the fog of pregnancy hormones descends. Topics can span the financial implications of childcare, parental leave, sharing baby care and household duties, and values related to how you actually want to raise your child.

Why do this now? Resentment is a huge issue for many couples. More women stay home to take care of their families than men,[1] and almost all women, regardless of their professional status, take on more chores. Even in families where both partners work, moms do the majority of scheduling, household labor, and stay home when children get sick. In the early days with an infant, especially if you're breastfeeding, an equitable division of baby care is not a realistic goal—unless men learn to lactate. But there are plenty of ways that your partner can contribute (sanitation crew, anyone?).

Pregnancy is the wildest transformation of most women's lives. At times, you won't feel, look, or even act like yourself. And no matter how marvelous or tuned-in your partner is, they will not completely understand the physical and emotional undertaking that is growing another human being. Instead of expecting psychic powers, tell them directly how to best support you, and be honest about how you're feeling. And ask them the same questions. Though they aren't living with the day-to-day of pregnancy, this is a big transition for them, too.

## PRECONCEPTION CHECKUP

If you already know whom you'd like to manage your prenatal care, now is a great time to schedule your first chat about improving your fertility and how to later have a healthy pregnancy. Not sure yet? Set an appointment with your current ob-gyn or gynecologist.

Partners, this is a wonderful time to schedule that long-overdue physical.

When you go in for an appointment, prepare for a slew of questions that will determine whether your pregnancy will require anything beyond standard-issue prenatal care, or extra steps during conception. Partners, you'll hear many of the same questions, especially related to lifestyle, family history, and genetic screenings.

Here are the questions you can expect:

- Age
- Family history
- Gynecological history (state of your period, current or past methods of birth control, STDs or abnormal Pap smears, history of infertility or past pregnancies)
- Medical history (chronic conditions, past surgeries or hospitalizations, exposure to infectious diseases)
- Medications and allergies (all prescription or OTC medications and supplements you are taking, including prenatal vitamins, and known allergies)
- Vaccinations (childhood history, Tdap [tetanus, diphtheria, acellular pertussis] vaccine, flu shot, and upcoming travel requiring vaccines)
- Lifestyle (profession; hobbies; relationship status; use of drugs, alcohol, tobacco, and caffeine; exercise, weight and dietary history)
- Emotional history (history of anxiety, depression or mood disorders, eating disorders, current or past domestic violence or sexual assault/rape)
- Genetic carrier screening (family history of birth defects, abnormalities, inherited disorders, miscarriages, or stillbirths)

Pending the answers, your physician may order tests if you have hormone-related issues, get you up-to-date with missing vaccines, and make lifestyle-related suggestions. The latter will definitely include cutting alcohol and caffeine consumption and putting a full stop to smoking and recreational drug use.

On that note, while it's tempting to downplay questionable behavior with your physician, now is not the time for half-truths. Studies show that women commonly conceal how much alcohol they consume, for example. If your practitioner is given incomplete or slightly fudged information, they can't provide the best care.

Partner, just because you won't be carrying the baby doesn't mean these rules don't apply to you, too. More and more data shows that men's behavior and habits impact sperm. Here are a few of the health and lifestyle factors that matter:

- Age (increased risk of chromosomal abnormalities over age forty)
- Smoking or vaping
- Drug and alcohol use (even cannabis, which changes sperm[2])
- Weight and diet
- Medications, including prescriptions, OTC treatments, and supplements
- Cancer treatments

Now back to you, ladies. Let's get real: Pregnancy is a weird time for your body. New medical problems can start, ongoing issues can get worse, and all of these changes can affect the safety and efficacy of medications you've taken for years.

Six out of every ten Americans have a chronic condition,[3] and four in ten have two or more. If you are in this large and growing pool, or take anything to manage your health, chat with your prescribing physician before trying to conceive.

Yes, partners, this means you, too. Some prescription drugs can impact sperm quality and quantity, so ideally, take care of this a few months before you start trying to conceive.

## FERTILITY TESTING

If you want even more insight into your reproductive health, there are a growing number of direct-to-consumer fertility tests on the market. The majority are available for under $300, and many can be purchased with your health savings account (HSA) or flexible spending account (FSA). Doing the same panel in-office with your doctor is not always covered by insurance, especially if it's coded as elective, meaning it can be much more expensive to get most of the same information with them.

These tests typically start with a quick physician phone screen. You'll volunteer a brief medical history, and will be directed to submit a blood sample via a finger prick from home, or by swinging by a local blood-draw center. The markers they test are related to ovarian reserves (the number and quality of available eggs in your ovaries) as well as ovulation and testosterone. The test results are emailed, or released during another phone consultation with a physician, who will walk you through the findings.

Partners, there are test kits for your swimmers, too. The process is similar, though the testing of sperm quality and quantity requires a different sort of contribution. There are basic versions available to do at home with instant results, or mail-in kits that provide more in-depth findings.

## GENETIC CARRIER SCREENINGS

Recalling the medical histories of every single family member and branch is challenging enough, even if you have access to those records. But some conditions don't present in every generation, so you also may not know about them.

Just in case you slept through high school biology, here is a crash course on the basics of genetic inheritance. After cultivating and testing thousands of pea plants, a monk named Gregor Mendel discovered that three basic principles applied to the passing of traits from parents to their offspring. Mendel's laws tl;dr: Offspring inherit one genetic marker from each parent independent of any others, and recessive markers will always be masked by those that are dominant.

A genetic carrier screening reveals whether you or your partner carry a genetic marker for any of a number of conditions, and how likely it is that your child will inherit it.[4] Done via blood draw, saliva sample, or cheek swab, it's noninvasive and tests primarily for cystic fibrosis, sickle cell disease, fragile X syndrome, and Tay-Sachs disease. Consumer-grade tests are available to order online, but if you think you might be at higher risk, it's best to do this screening through your physician.

Screenings start with full medical histories and testing the partner with higher carrier risk. The types of conditions your doctor may ask about are more varied, and you may not be as susceptible to some based on your background. If the results from the first partner's round of testing are clean, there is no need to do another, as it takes both of you for the condition to be an issue.

If you are both carriers for a serious condition, there are options. You can choose to get pregnant and rely on diagnostic tests to confirm whether your baby inherited the condition. IVF using your own sperm and eggs or donor gametes is another option. The fertilized embryos can be tested before implantation to ensure you will definitely not pass the condition down. A genetic counselor or your physician will guide this process, so you won't be making these decisions alone.

## EPIGENETICS

Could the way your parents or grandparents lived affect the way your baby processes stress? Epigenetics is the study of how lifestyle and health factors impact the inheritance and expression of traits without rewriting the actual DNA sequence, and shows how these changes could influence not only your child, but also the generations after.

Though the term *epigenetics* was first coined in 1940, we are only beginning to understand its implications. The research is fascinating, and reveals how much weight what we choose to do and put into our bodies carries. For example, it's no secret that the sons of moms who smoke during pregnancy have a lower sperm count. But smoking carries the same impact if Dad smoked, too, independent of Mom's actions. One study showed that the sons of fathers who smoked had 51 percent fewer sperm.[5]

So what are these health and lifestyle factors? They range from sleep patterns, exercise, age, and anxiety levels to where you live and whom you interact with. Epigenetic changes can also happen as a result of exposure to environmental factors like smoke, heavy metals, hormones, viruses, bacteria, and nutrients.[6]

If you're wondering, *Okay, so what do I do about it?* the answer is, like everything else related to pregnancy, file under "heard," and do the best you can to clean up your lifestyle. We simply don't know enough about epigenetics yet to say definitively if there are preventive measures or ways to reprogram these changes.

## *AU REVOIR* TO BIRTH CONTROL, AND GETTING TO KNOW YOUR CYCLE

Hormonal birth control works (for the most part) by stopping ovulation; no ovulation, no pregnancy. So if you're taking birth control or have an IUD, the first big step in downshifting to conception mode is to stop or take it out. If you're on the pill, you can quit whenever you want, though your bleeding schedule and ovulation may be irregular.

For long-term birth-control users, this can be a BIG transition. When you stop, expect some hormonal and mood changes. Gone will be the days of a light, predictable, symptom-free flow, if you were lucky enough to experience that. But good news: If birth control knocked down your libido, it may return once you stop.

The biggest change, however, is that with many formulations, you can get pregnant the very next cycle. The rhythm and pullout methods are not reliable, so be careful and use backup birth control if that is not your goal.

## Side effects of stopping birth control:

- Heavier periods
- Cramps
- Irregular cycle length
- Acne
- Weight fluctuations
- Fewer headaches

Exactly when a period will return in full force is different for everyone. Some come right back the first month. Others take longer. Once it does make an appearance, it's best to complete at least one full cycle before trying to conceive, to more accurately pinpoint your ovulation window. It also helps with more exact dating if you do get pregnant, as your due date is calculated based on the start of your last menstrual period (LMP).

Data points like your cycle length and blood volume and color in combination with a presence or lack of symptoms say a lot about the state of your fertility. We are all conditioned to think they are normal, but PMS symptoms like bloating, cramps, and acne are typically signs of hormonal imbalances. If yours are extreme, talk to your favorite practitioner or ob-gyn to debug.

Since you may be getting to know each other again, here are the basics of a normal, healthy menstrual cycle:

- **Full cycle length:** twenty-five to thirty-five days (a consistent duration month to month is more important than length)
- **Bleeding duration:** four to seven days

- **Color:** bright red (think cranberry juice) with no clots
- **Volume:** If you are filling up a tampon, pad, or cup in under four hours, it's likely too much and you should chat with your ob-gyn

Use your calendar or one of the many cycle-tracking apps to build a baseline. If your period is irregular or otherwise out of whack, look to diet and lifestyle first for simple tweaks. Stress, nutrition, exercise, and sleep all impact it, so try drinking more water and less caffeine and alcohol to start. It's normal to spot during ovulation, but if you have breakthrough bleeding outside of that time, take note and consult an ob-gyn.

*I was on the pill for almost twenty years to control cramping and digestive issues that started when I was a teenager, and I barely had any trace of a period. Most months, it didn't even occur to me that I had a period at all, since bleeding was so rare. When I quit, I expected a long lead time for my cycle to return normally, but was pleasantly surprised that it came back exactly twenty-eight days later.*

*My mood swings were a less pleasant surprise. Small things that normally didn't bother me, like dirty dishes in the sink, were all of a sudden a REALLY big deal. I was less touchy during pregnancy than in that first month off the pill.*

*We never expected to get pregnant the first time we tried, and on every subsequent attempt. Though our semi-crazy fertility hit rate is not typical, especially considering we are both in our mid-thirties, this is why I advocate for prepping your body in advance, since pregnancy can happen before you expect it.*

## PRENATAL VITAMINS

Eating a well-rounded, veggie-packed diet during pregnancy can be tough, especially if first-trimester morning sickness ensures that all you can choke down is crackers. Combined with its proven reduction in neural tube[7] and heart defects, preterm birth,[8] low birth weights, and even autism, the magical prenatal vitamin is key from conception through breastfeeding.

The benefits of folic acid, the powerhouse ingredient in prenatal vitamins, were first published by the British hematologist Lucy Wills in 1931.[9] She noticed that poor pregnant workers in India suffered from anemia at much higher rates than the wealthy, and tied it to nutrition. She successfully treated these women with liver supplements and Marmite (a salty paste made from yeast extract that's all the rage in the UK), both of which share a high concentration of vitamin B9. And so it was that the "Wills Factor," or folic acid, was heralded as a breakthrough in the treatment of nutritional anemias.

Folic acid is the synthetic form of vitamin B9 found in processed foods and most supplements, and still powers the prenatal vitamins we take today. Folate is the naturally occurring version found in foods like eggs, leafy greens, avocado, and liver. Refined grains are enriched with folic acid, so cereal, flour, and pasta in concert with folate-packed kale help, but are not enough to allow you to skip prenatal vitamins.

The ideal time to start taking prenatal vitamins is three months before you try to conceive so levels can build up in your system. When you go shopping, here are the top ingredients to seek out on the label:

- Folic acid (5-MTHF is a great choice if available)
- Iron
- Calcium
- Vitamin D
- Iodine
- Omega-3 fatty acids (DHA and EPA)

Though side effects are usually minimal, the iron in prenatal vitamins can cause stomach issues or nausea, so take them at night before you go to bed, with a snack, or look for food-based versions that are easier to digest.

One last biology lesson, this time on the MTHFR gene mutation (it doesn't stand for what you think it does). The MTHFR gene tells your body how to make the enzyme methylenetetrahydrofolate reductase, otherwise known as MTHFR.[10] When you eat food or take supplements containing folic acid, MTHFR converts it into methylfolate, the active format your body can actually use. With the MTHFR mutation, your body cannot properly convert and then absorb folate or folic acid. It is also thought to affect hormones, digestion, cholesterol, and brain function, and may be a cause of recurrent miscarriage.

Carriers of the MTHFR gene are typically asymptomatic. For that reason, medical groups don't suggest routine testing. If you know you have the mutation, talk to your doctor and choose a prenatal vitamin with the active, already methalyzed form of folic acid, methylfolate (L-methylfolate, L-5-methyltetrahydrofolate, or L-5-MTHF), listed on the label.

## ZIKA

Birth defects are reported in roughly 3 percent of US births[11] each year. Though it gets a lot of media exposure, Zika is responsible for very few of them. In fact, even if you have Zika while pregnant, there is no guarantee that your baby will be born with issues. Just 5 to 10 percent of confirmed Zika infections during pregnancy are associated with birth defects,[12] and the risk is highest if the infection happens during the first trimester.

So what is Zika anyway? It is a virus that causes birth defects like microcephaly (a condition that causes an abnormally small head). It is typically contracted through mosquito bites, but can also be sexually transmitted. Common symptoms include joint pain, eye in-flammation, fever, and rash. If you're worried about an infection, lab testing can confirm a diagnosis.

Even though the Zika threat has been downgraded, the effects of an infection while you are pregnant are serious, especially since there is no approved treatment or vaccine. To avoid it, sadly, you and your partner should avoid travel to places where it's active. Check the Centers for Disease Control and Prevention (CDC) website for up-to-date guidance on specific destinations. If you are planning to visit a place with active Zika, the guideline is to wait six to eight weeks for the virus to clear your system before trying to conceive. However, Zika can remain in sperm for up to six months. So if your partner has traveled to an active Zika area, or knows he's had Zika, it's recommended that you wait those six months before trying to conceive, and use protection if you are already pregnant.

## FINANCES

Getting a handle on your health and getting pregnant is only part of the "having a kid" equation. The other major component? Money.

The United States is the priciest place in the world to give birth. An uncomplicated vaginal delivery is more expensive than the British royal family's private luxury births, costing over $10,000 on average.[13] That price jumps to over $30,000 when you add prenatal and postnatal care. Though having insurance helps bring down out-of-pocket costs, plans vary widely when it comes to maternity care, so you should be prepared to spend several thousand dollars outside of your monthly premiums even if things go smoothly.

What about after? Raising a child from birth to age seventeen costs about $233,610[14] for middle-income families. This does not include a college education, nor does it account for indirect costs like your time, lost earnings, or missed career opportunities. In the first years of life, the biggest financial outlays are housing and childcare. Full-time day care is roughly $10,000 per year—much more in coastal cities—and a full-time nanny is about $30,000.[15]

In other words, having a kid is not cheap. Exact expenses vary depending on where you live, but these high costs, especially childcare, come as a surprise to three of every four new parents. Three-quarters of expectant parents assume childcare costs won't impact their career decisions, but 63 percent report later that they did.

There are tax credits available for families, and contributing to a Dependent Care Flexible Spending Account is another money-saving option, but support from the government or your employer is not a reality for most US families. Though childcare remains one of the most highly sought-after benefits from employers, only one in five currently offers it.

The surprise costs of having children can also have unsavory effects on a couple's emotional well-being. A study spanning thirty-five countries, eight years, and over a million people[16] showed that having kids lowered happiness until you controlled for the ability to pay your bills. For couples who plan for these costs, building a family is more likely to be a universal positive.

How you divide and manage financial responsibilities is unique to your individual careers, your relationship dynamic, and how you visualize the first few years of your child's life. The earlier you plan and talk about this together, the more prepared you will be to handle surprises, and the less likely you are to fight later.

Humans successfully raised children for thousands of years before BabyBjörn. So while outfitting a nursery and accessorizing your baby can be expensive, you can minimize those optional costs. To start a baby budget, look at your current finances, available savings, and monthly burn rate. The two major pregnancy line items not wholly under your control are medical expenses and childcare, so begin researching and planning those costs before diving into the fun stuff.

Here are the inputs and discussions that will inform your budget:

- Research your insurance plan (the next section will help with what to ask) to see how much prenatal and birth care is covered in time to make changes to your plan. If you don't have insurance, see if there's a way to enroll on your partner's plan, or through the exchange.
- Talk about what type of childcare (if any) will be necessary after birth when and if you go back to work or need an extra hand.
- Most parents who stock up on clothes, toys, and gadgets before getting to know their baby's preferences will tell you they should have waited. Save money by purchasing items like cribs and cots used, borrow as many basics as you can, and remember that although you need a lot of them, kitchen towels work just as well as specialty burp cloths.
- The biggest ongoing infant expenses are diapers and, if you aren't breastfeeding, formula (though breastfeeding isn't free either). Standard issue, non-specialty versions of both cost more than $1,200 per year.
- You'll wear maternity clothes for only a few months, so look in your closet for pieces with extra room at the waistband or that will stretch to accommodate your growing belly, borrow, buy used, or rent before you invest in a spendy pregnancy wardrobe.

## INSURANCE

Don't shut the book. I know, this isn't the fun stuff, and navigating the ins and outs of insurance coverage is about as fun as finding the exit in a Vegas casino. In this case, however, there is a payoff—literally.

Reviewing your coverage before you actually get pregnant allows you to check whether your desired birth spot, practitioners, and pre/post services (if you have already chosen these things) are included. Hard costs like deductibles, copays, and out-of-pocket maxes will also help you build a realistic budget. If open enrollment happens during those nine long months, you can upgrade to access new services and cut your out-of-pocket maximum. How much you pay out of pocket depends entirely on the details of your plan. Generally, the higher the premium, the lower the deductible and out-of-pocket costs. The only way to know for sure is to look up the specifics.

Pro tip: Pregnancy is not a "qualifying life event" that allows you to change your coverage outside of open enrollment periods—but birth is. In the thirty to sixty days after the baby pops out, you can add Junior and make further changes to your plan. Upgrading or downgrading afterward will not affect costs related to birth. However, if you decided to go premium while pregnant and want to move to a less expensive plan when you're done, it's possible to do so. Just consider the five to seven pediatrician appointments in your baby's first year of life before you cut, as costs for vaccinations and those visits add up.

So what's generally covered by insurance?

- Pre- and postnatal doctor's appointments, labs, medications, and treatments or screenings for conditions like diabetes
- Inpatient experiences including birth, hospitalizations, and assorted hospital fees
- Breast pump and lactation counseling
- Newborn-baby care (shots and tests done in the hospital, vaccines, well-baby visits)

Another huge benefit of understanding your insurance is that you may discover unexpected and cool services that are partially or even fully covered. Again, depending on your plan, these might include acupuncture, physical therapy, a doula, massage, or 24/7 video access to nurses and other health professionals. For those wondering what on earth a doula is, we'll get there. Yes, visiting complementary practitioners can mean paying up front and submitting claims afterward, which is annoying. But bonus: Navigating that gauntlet is a *fabulous* activity for your partner while you are busy baking your tiny human.

One last thing: Pregnancy is a perfect time to spend those stored FSA (flexible spending account) or HSA (health savings account) dollars. If these accounts are new concepts, think of them as savings accounts built with pretax dollars funneled directly from your paycheck. Spend them on copays, deductibles, prenatal vitamins, baby-related medical items, or postpartum items for you. If you really run out of ideas, you can always stock up on sunscreen. Talk to HR to get one set up if it's available at your company or your partner's.

## WORK

This is the first of several sad reminders that policies supporting families and the health of new mothers are fairly nonexistent in the US today, which is why planning ahead is so critical.

Seventy-five percent of American moms with children under eighteen are employed full-time.[17] They are the primary or sole earners for 40 percent of families, yet the United States is the only developed country with no government-sponsored or employer-mandated paid parental leave policy.[18] It's not that way for the rest of the world. Canadian mothers get a full year of paid leave after having a baby. The UK grants thirty-nine weeks. In Finland, it's *three years*.

It took until 1993 for the US to approve up to twelve weeks of *unpaid* leave for each parent through the Family and Medical Leave Act (FMLA). The act requires health benefits be maintained during leave and entitles employees to return to the same or equivalent job afterward. It does not, however, mandate any pay. Though some states and cities have policies to support new families financially, the majority of the responsibility falls squarely on employers.

That responsibility is taken on by only 14 percent of US companies, and access is stratified.[19] The highest-income workers are 3.5 times more likely to have this benefit than those in the lowest-income positions. Even in highly paid sectors like technology, finance, science, insurance, and other professional services, less than half of companies provide parental leave.

The advantages of parental leave for businesses are proven. Women who take paid leave are over 90 percent more likely to be in the workforce a year after birth than those who don't. And employee retention isn't the only reward. Good family policies also help attract talent, improve a company's brand, and even increase productivity. Given all of this, the number of businesses that provide family benefits is slowly growing.

If you or your partner are lucky enough to have employee-sponsored leave, knowing what to expect financially is much easier. If not, what you're entitled to differs based on the size of your employer and how long you've been working there, as you have to qualify[20] to receive FMLA benefits.

Here are the broad strokes: If you work at a public agency or a private-sector company that has employed fifty or more people for at least a year, your employer has to participate. But (there's always a but!) even if your company is covered, your individual tenure must be at least twelve months—and 1,250 hours—prior to leave.

Confused yet? Here's a cheat code. If you work at a large company full-time, maternity and paternity leave policies will be spelled out in your HR handbook, so start there before trying to decipher the Department of Labor's muddle of information. Same deal if you work for the government or a public institution full-time. If you work at a small company, especially one employing fewer than fifty people, it's trickier, as they are not covered by FMLA rules, and may not yet have set policies. Working part-time may disqualify you from any benefits no matter where you work.

Though financial and life planning may seem like the least sexy part of the conception process, feeling more financially secure while trying to conceive will reduce your stress, which improves your odds of getting pregnant. And planning can ensure the whole having-a-family thing continues to be a positive for you and your partner, and that you are prepared (as much as anyone can be!) for whatever comes your way.

## #PARENTINGGOALS

We assume everyone building a family is ready for it. But not all pregnancies are planned! Here's a secret: Even the most relaxed, assured-looking parents who plan for years have moments, especially when faced with an inconsolable newborn at 3 a.m.

A big mental hurdle for most first-time mothers and fathers is deciding who they are and how they want to show up in the world as parents. This identity is tied to so many things—your age, your professional experience, how you perceive gender roles and responsibilities, your own childhood, and your financial resources, just to name a few.

Start by asking yourself why you want to have a child, and if you have a specific idea of what your future family will look like. There is no right answer, just what feels right to you. Then consider what kind of parent you'd like to be. Share with your significant other and see how their personal vision overlaps with yours. Even if you've talked about it before, you might find there are areas where you diverge now that it's all becoming real.

Everyone enters parenting as someone else's child. We learn habits and behaviors from our parents, which affect the way we approach our own time as parents. Your upbringing does not dictate who you become, but can have unintended side effects if you don't take the time to digest it. Whether your childhood was complicated or great or somewhere in between, try to reflect on who your parents are, why they did what they did, and how it affected you. Kudos if you've already covered this in therapy. If it's still difficult, it may be worth recruiting some professional help to process.

Ready to start practicing co-parenting and communication? Take a few minutes several times a week to check in with each other. Talk about your days, about what's working at home, what's not, and what needs to change. If you're not always face-to-face, this can also happen asynchronously via text or messenger or video. If you wait to form these habits until an infant is around, they probably won't stick. As time goes on, these conversations will evolve, as will your individual and shared identities.

When your new addition does finally make his or her appearance, keep the lines of communication open and share your parenting philosophy with others, especially caregivers, family, and friends. If you have a specific value system or set of principles, it's important to be surrounded by others who share (or are at least willing to adhere to) them.

Figuring out what doesn't work is just as important as discovering what does, and effort goes a long way even when you make mistakes. And you will make mistakes—every new parent does. Kids have a baseline that you can't always control, and your relationship with them shouldn't always be about discipline. We listen to people we trust, so through consistency and flexibility, you can help your children trust you.

# YOUR CARE TEAM
# FANTASY DRAFT

## Recruiting the perfect practitioners
## to manage your pregnancy

**B**efore you meet the bevy of amazing humans who can help steer your pregnancy, let's see how we got here.

From the landing of the *Mayflower* to revolutionary times, childbirth in the US was a community event.[1] Women received advice and help from friends and family during labor. Men were not part of childbirth; in fact, there were laws in some places that actually forbade their involvement, as it was considered scandalous even in a medical context for any man other than a woman's husband to see her in a state of undress. It wasn't until the 1970s that fathers were widely admitted to the delivery room at all.

Midwives led nearly all deliveries, and were held in high social regard. But around the time the ink was drying on the Constitution in 1787, the inevitable social stratification of childbirth began. A new range of options allowed women to buy a better experience, and the rise of American medical schools led to more formalized education for physicians. This training was offered only to men, so the primarily female midwives of the age missed out, and "male midwives," or the first obstetricians, replaced them.

The result was a big departure from the nurturing cadre of fellow mothers and ladies. In this more authoritative model, modesty and privacy were status symbols, prized above emotional support.

Midwives had no formal organization to represent their interests as physicians did. Ads portrayed them as witch doctors driven only by money, in stark contrast to the physician's image as safe and trustworthy. And it worked. Many states banned midwifery completely, or made it logistically impossible for midwives to practice.

The shift really solidified after Dr. Joseph DeLee, considered the founder of modern obstetrics, started the Chicago Lying-In Hospital in 1917.[2] His improvement of hygienic practices and a medicalized approach to childbirth yielded a maternal mortality rate 25 percent of the national average, which was significant, considering an average of one in every 154 women died during birth. His innovations included the first portable incubator and fetoscope, and separate facilities and laundry for birthing as preventive measures against hospital-acquired infection.

DeLee was no fan of midwifery, and did further public damage to its reputation. He believed that the practice lowered the "dignity of obstetric art and science"[3] and found fault with its community roots. He also decried the lack of training and professionalism. His view was that all women, regardless of financial status, should have access to the same medical care, and that this single standard should be obstetrics.

While his improvements saved lives and formed the foundation for many of today's medical practices, DeLee's interventionist approach had less positive effects on obstetric care, too. One of his legacies was the use of forceps and episiotomy (an incision made in the perineum to enlarge the vaginal opening during childbirth), even when there were no complications that required mechanical intervention. Forty percent of babies born vaginally in the US in the early 1970s were delivered with forceps, and 90 percent of mothers received an episiotomy. Thankfully, research proved that these practices should be exercised only if medically indicated; the episiotomy rate dropped to below 20 percent by 2000 and continues to decline. Leapfrog, a national nonprofit patient safety organization, set a target goal of a 5 percent episiotomy rate, and many hospitals now meet that metric.

Today we're seeing a move back to less intervention and the reemergence of midwives as part of a coordinated care team across all birth settings. Midwives increasingly participate alongside doctors at hospitals, and lead nearly all birth-center and at-home births.

So where do births happen in the US today? Though less than 2 percent take place outside hospitals, that number is on the rise. Only 1 percent occur at home, which is a low percentage compared to the rest of the world. The number of birth centers in the US has risen by over 80 percent in the past decade[4] to fill the growing demand.

The main reason the out-of-hospital birth rate is so low? Risk. As many as one-third of all first-time mothers who attempt at-home births transfer to the hospital anyway,[5] and babies die at twice the rate during home births as they do in hospitals. The admission rate drops to 9 percent for those who have given birth before, making it a better option for subsequent kids. If you're considering it, home births are appropriate only in low-risk pregnancies with informed consent so that you understand the risks, and involve practitioners trained in neonatal resuscitation. Geographically, it's ideal for home births to take place within a fifteen-minute drive of a hospital just in case.

Standard prenatal visits cannot cover everything, which is why more diverse teams are necessary to help pregnant women manage their minds and bodies outside the clinical setting. There are tremendous benefits to maintaining a strong pelvic floor, understanding the role of nutrition, and managing mental health issues; ways to improve birth outcomes through the care of doulas; and nonmedical practices like acupuncture, bodywork, and massage that can help you stay comfortable and relaxed. A growing number of apps and products put these practices within reach no matter how busy you find yourself, and reduce their costs.

Some of the professionals we'll explore in this section, like ob-gyns, will be familiar to you, while others, like doulas, may be new. Though you won't engage with some until later in your pregnancy, it's helpful to understand how and when they provide value, and what, if anything, insurance covers.

If time is your most precious resource, and the idea of scheduling anything other than prenatal appointments feels like too much, have no fear. Telemedicine and services with more flexibility are included, too, and are accessible from wherever, whenever.

Pregnancy and childbirth, as you likely have already noticed, are not zero-sum. Rather than adhere to a specific ideology or framework, create your own as you go along. And be prepared to pivot as necessary!

## PRENATAL CARE PROVIDERS

The first specialist to choose in your fantasy draft is the quarterback for your prenatal care. The two most common options are ob-gyns and midwives. If you have a high-risk pregnancy, or are managing a chronic condition (like hypertension or diabetes), starting with an ob-gyn is standard, though you may be able to transition to a midwife later if everything progresses normally. If your pregnancy is sans complications, a midwife can be the main point of contact during most of your prenatal care. This goes for planned home births and those taking place in birthing centers and, increasingly, in hospital settings. In fact, a growing number of hospitals now have midwives on staff and present during birth, regardless of who manages your prenatal care.

It can be overwhelming to know where to start unless you have a referral from friends, or already have a practitioner you like. If you're struggling, start by thinking about your ideal birth experience. For example, if you want to deliver at a center and not a hospital, you'll need to find a practitioner, most likely a midwife, approved to practice at that facility. If you have a specific hospital in mind, ensure that your ob-gyn has rights to practice there. If you have options, investigate the cesarean section rate at the hospital you're considering, as rates can vary between 7 and 70 percent. Next up: Call your insurance provider to see what and whom they cover. At-home births and birth centers are rarely covered by insurance, so you'll likely be on the hook for those costs.

### Ob-gyns

Nearly all births in the US happen in a hospital, and are led or assisted by an obstetrician-gynecologist. The term *obstetrics* refers to childbirth, and gynecology deals with the reproductive health conditions specific to women and girls. Fun fact: Not all gynecologists are obstetricians, but all obstetricians are gynecologists, so if your physician lacks the "ob" in front of the "gyn," it's time to find someone who doesn't.

An ob-gyn's practice may be in a traditional office setting or a hospital. Specialists in these practices include not only the ob-gyns themselves, but often nurse practitioners, midwives, sonographers, dietitians, genetic counselors, social workers, lactation consultants, and physician assistants. Your exposure to each subspecialty will depend on the specifics of your pregnancy and your desire to enlist additional help.

Choosing the right ob-gyn is important, as they will be your sherpa through this long, often confusing, and very personal process. However, it's helpful to remember two critical facts about this relationship.

**Fact #1:** Though you will see this person with increasing frequency toward the end of your pregnancy, your total time together amounts to only a handful of hours, especially if you are low risk. You'll see your provider once per month in the first and second trimesters, once every two weeks in the third trimester up to thirty-six weeks, and once per week from thirty-six weeks through pop time. Here is a snapshot view of a standard prenatal appointment and testing schedule:

| Time | Action |
|------|--------|
| 8–10 weeks | First appointment and ultrasound (you'll also learn your due date!) |
| 10–12 weeks | Initial blood draw for first health screening and non-invasive prenatal testing (NIPT) if requested |
| 12 weeks | Nuchal translucency measurement ultrasound and genetic counseling (if NIPT testing was requested) |
| 16 weeks | Blood tests and prenatal checkup |
| 18–20 weeks | Anatomy scan ultrasound (you'll find out gender if you don't already know!) and prenatal checkup |
| 24 weeks | Glucose screening for gestational diabetes and prenatal checkup |
| 28 weeks | Prenatal checkup |
| 32 weeks | Final ultrasound (typically only done in higher-risk pregnancies) and prenatal checkup |
| 36 weeks | Prenatal checkup |
| 38 weeks | Prenatal checkup |
| 39 weeks | Prenatal checkup |
| 40 weeks | Prenatal checkup |
| 41 weeks | Induction if labor hasn't started on its own |
| 1–6 weeks postpartum | If you had high blood pressure during pregnancy, you'll need a checkup within a week of leaving the hospital. Otherwise, a follow-up appointment at six weeks postpartum is normal. |

Each prenatal appointment will include a Q&A session for you, a weight measurement and blood pressure reading, a discussion of any new medications or issues since the previous appointment, a chance to listen to your baby's heartbeat, measurement of your belly (from the second trimester on), a mental health check-in, and any additional tests due that week.

**Fact #2:** A few private practitioners still attend each of their patients' births, but in general, the days of ob-gyns on call are over. And it's a good thing for patient care, as there are high burnout rates associated with the stress of the job.

There's always a chance you'll see a new face in the delivery room, as schedules change, and many hospitals now employ a laborist model powered by a rotating group of practitioners called OB hospitalists. Think of them as a hospital's commitment to safety, as they are focused solely on childbirth and obstetrical emergencies. They work only in the hospital and do not typically provide prenatal care, so your odds of seeing them before birth are slim.

Practically speaking, this means that it's unlikely the doctor you've poured out every concern and ache and pain to during prenatal visits will be the one to actually deliver your baby. If you have strong feelings, ask about the practice's care model before or during your first prenatal visit, then find someone who is willing to be on call. Setting appointments throughout your pregnancy with different ob-gyns to get to know everyone is another tactic to increase the odds of a friendly face at your delivery.

### Things to consider when choosing an ob-gyn

If you need to choose someone new, here are a few questions to answer before and during that first appointment:

- Are they in-network for my insurance?
- What is their hospital affiliation, and where would I deliver?

- If my physician isn't the one to deliver, who will be?
- How does my doctor feel about my preferred birth and pain medication preferences?
- Does the doctor have a good bedside manner?
- What about the rest of the staff?
- What is their C-section rate and episiotomy rate, and do they perform VBACs? (VBAC = vaginal birth after C-section)

*As a member of the dreaded over-thirty-five, advanced-maternal-age crew, I was in the high-risk category, thanks to my "elderly" status; this meant I saw a special type of ob-gyn called a perinatologist for my prenatal care. When I realized I would probably not see her in the delivery room, I booked appointments with the other practitioners who might show up. All of them had slightly different styles, and I learned a lot seeing a wider range of people.*

*Because I knew in advance that this is how things work, I did not feel any attachment to who was present when I actually gave birth. And I was glad I made my peace with it, as an OB hospitalist led my delivery, assisted by a team of residents I'd never set eyes on before.*

### Midwives

Midwifery suffers from a serious branding problem. Many still assume that midwives, long marked as grandmas in the woods, serve only at home births and do not have formal medical training. While some are based in birthing centers and, yes, supervise at-home births, a growing number are hospital-based and practice alongside ob-gyns.

Today's midwives receive rigorous medical training (in fact, many have master's degrees) and can prescribe medication. They can manage care throughout pregnancy, birth, and postpartum, primarily in low-risk pregnancies, though they can manage more complicated births under ob-gyn supervision.

If you're trying to choose, outside of medical training, the biggest difference in care between an ob-gyn and a midwife is the experience. Ob-gyn visits are more focused on tests, metrics, and clinical care. Midwives generally spend more time with patients, focus less on interventions and more on unmedicated birthing options, and cater to the emotional side of pregnancy. Like ob-gyn practices, most hospital-based midwifery practices also operate in a cohort model, which means you may see a variety of practitioners during your pregnancy and there's no way of guaranteeing which one will be at the birth.

There are three different certification levels and abilities for midwives. The main difference is the type of training they receive and whether they have a nursing certification.

**Certified nurse-midwives (CNMs)** are the type you are most likely to encounter in a traditional medical setting, as they are licensed registered nurses who go on to earn a certification from the American College of Nurse-Midwives. Some CNMs perform home births and practice at birthing centers, but the majority work alongside ob-gyns in private or hospital settings. They can provide the full spectrum of prenatal care, and most can write prescriptions.

**Certified midwives (CMs)** are most relevant if you live in Delaware, Missouri, New Jersey, New York, or Rhode Island, where they are licensed to practice, and take the same exam as CNMs. The main difference: Though their graduate-level education and testing are the same, they do not have a nursing degree.

**Certified professional midwives (CPMs)** are best if you are giving birth at home or in a birth center, as these practitioners are required to be experienced in both. Training is less standardized than for CMs and CNMs, and they are generally not licensed nurses. The North American Registry of Midwives (NARM) provides the certification for this group.

There can be challenges to working with a midwife. The first:

state-by-state rules that dictate the limits of their practice, and whether they are allowed to practice at all. (Ironically, the states with the most restrictive policies also have the highest rates of adverse birth outcomes!)

There is also the issue of paying for it. Medicaid is obligated to cover midwifery services, but private insurance often lacks in-network providers or refuses to cover it at all. An uncomplicated vaginal birth in a hospital costs over $10,000. Similar births outside the hospital cost half that. While that out-of-pocket expenditure may be out of reach for many parents, the potential cost savings to the healthcare system are significant.

Midwives attend just 8 percent of US births today, but the benefits of reintegrating them back into the healthcare system go beyond money. Hospital births supervised by midwives are less likely to end in a C-section or other medical intervention, and the high-touch model can be much more emotionally fulfilling than traditional clinical care.

*While I did not manage my prenatal care with a midwife, there was one at my birth. My experience was very positive, and made me wish my pregnancy was low risk so I could have mixed in a few visits with her. She was an oasis of calm, and gently coached me through contractions and provided practical advice and ways to manage pain.*

### Family practice physicians

If you already see someone you love for everyday issues and are low risk, it's fine to start prenatal care with your family-practice physician. The main benefit to this provider type is they already know you and your medical history, and can later take on the role of pediatrician when your baby comes along.

However, their training is focused on a range of medical conditions, not obstetrics specifically, so most are not equipped to handle high-risk pregnancies. If you run into any complications, they will have to refer you to an ob-gyn, and may not be the one to handle labor and delivery.

### Group prenatal care

Hospitals and private medical practices also offer group prenatal care, which brings together pregnant women due around the same time. You'll still have a relationship with a physician or midwife, but care is not constrained to short individual exams. Instead, each session is about sixty to ninety minutes and includes your prenatal appointment and a group discussion. Studies have shown improved pregnancy outcomes with this care model.

Another benefit most new parents cite is making friends who are in the same life stage. Some even stage reunions, or pool childcare resources. Like working with a midwife, group care is generally utilized in low-risk pregnancies, though it's possible to take advantage of both individual appointments and a group setting if you want the additional support.

## COMPLEMENTARY PRACTITIONERS

### Doulas

Translated from Greek, the word *doula* literally means "woman's servant." That meaning holds true in English, too. Doulas are health professionals who provide emotional, physical, and educational support to you and your partner before, during, and after birth. This support ranges from knowing when it's time to go to the hospital and coaching you (and your partner) through birth, to help with breastfeeding afterward. They cannot prescribe drugs, diagnose health conditions, or perform clinical procedures, as few have medical backgrounds.

In 2006, just 3 percent of parents used a doula during childbirth. By 2012, this number had doubled; it continues to climb today. That's a good thing, as women with continuous support during labor are more likely to have spontaneous vaginal births and shorter labor. They are also less likely to have C-sections, and have a lower need for pain medication. Their babies have higher Apgar scores (the test done right after birth to quickly summarize a newborn's health) and less trouble breastfeeding. In general, everyone also leaves the birth experience feeling more positive.[6]

Labor can be long, especially in a first birth, and if it is, there may be stretches of time when you and your partner will be left alone. Labor and delivery nurses are amazing, but they often have more than one patient, and their priority is to provide clinical care. Same for midwives and OBs. Doulas are not hospital employees—they are there just for you. And they are just as valuable to your partner (in some cases even more so), even if only to give them an occasional break.

Your relationship starts at the beginning of the third trimester and lasts through the first weeks postpartum. Pre-birth meetings focus on understanding your needs, creating birth preferences, and teaching your partner how to be part of the labor process. Many doulas are also childbirth educators; in fact, some even lead the classes taught at hospitals. When it comes time for birth, they will be on call during early labor, then join you at home until it's go time. At the hospital or birth center, they will help you relax, practice nonmedical pain relief techniques, and be your advocate if needed. After your baby arrives, most doulas hang around to help with breastfeeding, and visit after you return home. Some even provide ongoing support through the first year of your infant's life.

The main credentialing organization for doulas is DONA International, but there are others popping up as the popularity of the practice rises. Though certification and experience are important, just as critical are trust and whether you feel at ease in their company. Things get pretty intimate during birth (perineal heating pads, anyone?), so be comfortable with the idea of your doula touching and coaching you during the intensity of labor.

Some doulas have strong opinions about the use of interventions, C-sections, and the appropriate scope of medical care, so understanding their birth philosophy is important, too. Their job is not to tell you how to give birth, or to overrule your physician. It's to determine your values, provide information, and answer questions, then support you in whatever birthing process you choose. If you're giving birth at a hospital, let your physician know you're planning to hire a doula at a prenatal appointment so they can note it in your chart. There can be tension between medical professionals and doulas, often relieved through communication.

A referral from a friend or healthcare provider or fitness studio that teaches prenatal classes is another great way to find a doula. If you're starting cold, Dona.org has a database of their certified practitioners to search. Find a few options, then interview several doulas to see what style and approach is right for you. Include your partner in these discussions, since they will spend just as much time with the doula as you will. The time to start looking for a doula is in the second trimester, as many of them book up far in advance.

Here are a few questions to ask during the interview process:

- Where did you receive your labor support training? Do you have any additional certifications or training?
- How many births have you attended and how long have you been practicing?
- What are your values and goals in providing your services to families?
- What is your approach to interactions with a medical team? Do you typically practice in hospitals?
- How do you handle long births? Do you leave to sleep/take breaks?
- What kind of support do you provide for partners?

- Can you share an outline of the visits we'll have before and after birth?
- How many clients do you take each month?
- What happens when I go into labor? What kind of support do you provide?
- What if labor happens before or after my due date and you are not available? Do you work in a team? How many times have you needed a backup doula?
- What are your fees and what is included?

Insurance rarely covers a doula's services. Out of pocket, their fees can range from $400 to $2,500, depending on their experience and your geography. Some state healthcare programs are looking at reimbursement, especially in low-income populations, thanks to the 41 percent reduction in C-sections when doulas are present,[7] but it's still rare.

*I'm going to get a little gushy now. My husband, Nick, and I could not imagine having gone through our birth without our doula team, especially considering, as you'll see later, it didn't go at all as we expected. They were the best investment we made during pregnancy. Besides teaching our birth class; providing text support, coaching, and hairbrushing during sixty-plus hours of labor; advocating for me when things got complicated; giving Nick breaks; and performing postpartum check-ins, they were lovely humans to boot.*

*I could keep going but you get the picture. This is why personally, I'm very excited to see doulas become more integrated into the birth experience and call on insurance companies and states to provide reimbursement or pay for their services.*

## *Acupuncture*

If you associate acupuncture only with pain relief, stress, and hippies, you're not alone—but you are missing out.

Acupuncture is a branch of Chinese medicine that uses thin needles to stimulate specific points on the body. Depending on where the needles are placed, you might feel relaxed or energized, or experience localized effects in one area.

We don't know exactly why or how acupuncture works. It may inspire the body to produce endorphins, the hormones that provide natural pain relief. It's possible that it stimulates the nervous system or changes how pain is perceived.[8]

If you rely on anecdotes and early research, there are reasons to get excited about acupuncture's positive effects on reproductive health. Due to its effects on the hypothalamus-pituitary-ovarian (HPO) axis, it is used to improve hormone-related problems. The HPO axis is responsible for production of FSH (follicle-stimulating hormone), which stimulates ovarian follicles to grow and mature, and LH (luteinizing hormone), which stimulates ovulation. Targeted treatments have shown promise in dealing with problem periods,[9] endometriosis, PCOS (polycystic ovary syndrome), and other menstrual issues.

Acupuncture is used differently throughout pregnancy. During conception, it can help send blood and oxygen to the reproductive organs, impacting the quality of the eggs maturing before ovulation. During the three trimesters of pregnancy it can diminish many of the annoying aches[10] and symptoms. It is used to stimulate labor and, during labor, to reduce pain. Postpartum, it can help rebalance hormones.

If you want to give it a whirl, look for clinics that specialize in fertility or women's health. Expect a suggested schedule of once per week during conception through the first trimester, then as needed in the second and third trimesters. Already seeing a reproductive endocrinologist? They may suggest acupuncture as a complementary practice, especially if you are receiving IUI (intrauterine insemination) or IVF (in vitro fertilization) treatments.

Appointments begin with a general status update, check-in on existing or new symptoms, and specific goals for your treatment. Acupuncturists receive training across many modalities of Chinese medicine, so they'll also suggest lifestyle and nutrition modifications, especially consumption of warm cooked foods like bone broth and congee. After the needle insertion you'll be left for fifteen to forty-five minutes so the treatment can do its magic. It's a great time for an epic cat nap, as the points acupuncture targets also help you to relax.

The average cost per appointment depends on your geography but is typically $75 to $150. Many practices accept insurance, which means you'll have a copay or be reimbursed for the full treatment cost later. Call your insurance company to ensure they preapprove treatments, and that the provider you're seeing is in network.

*I'll admit I was skeptical the first time I tried acupuncture to help with a sports injury. Especially as I am not great (okay, fine—I'm terrible) with needles and expected it to hurt, or that I would leave my appointment feeling like a pincushion. But it didn't hurt, and was more effective pain relief than anything my doctor prescribed.*

*After hearing friends sing acupuncture's praises in regard to conception, I decided to try it. While it's unclear whether it had a definitive impact on my fertility (possible, since I went to weekly appointments all three times we conceived), the main benefit it provided was helping me through the rough patches. Having a weekly check-in with my practitioner followed by a relaxing break eased a lot of my anxiety and provided the emotional support I didn't even know I needed. The appointment cadence changed based on my schedule, but I found treatments most valuable for whatever oomph it gave*

*our conception odds, recovery between pregnancies, and in*
*handling first-trimester discomfort and blahs.*

### Therapists

Pregnancy is supposed to be the happiest time of your life, right? Friends and family are excited, and you're sporting a gorgeous pregnant glow and on the cusp of welcoming a brand-new life that *you* created in *your* body from scratch. Isn't that beautiful? How could anyone need therapy at such a perfectly lovely time?

As you've probably figured out by now, the journey to becoming a parent isn't always sunshine and puppies. Sometimes it's *hard*. Even if it's relatively painless, it's a huge personal transformation. Your identity changes. Your hormones change. Your body changes. Your partnership changes. Your professional life, finances, and responsibilities do, too. Some of these changes are great. Some less so.

Talking to your pumped-up inner circle on the down days can feel off-limits in the face of so much enthusiasm. Which is why having an impartial third party around is so helpful.

Therapy isn't just for when things go wrong. Nor does it have to involve lying on a couch dissecting your relationship with your mother. Or father. Or ex-boyfriend. Therapy is unfairly associated only with people who are unhappy or dealing with a clinical condition when in fact, it's valuable when applied to life transitions and utilized for smaller periods of time, too.

Four in five women report mood changes associated with pregnancy and postpartum, and one in five women report depression or anxiety during pregnancy and postpartum. Even that number is believed to be wildly underreported. So if you're reading this and thinking, *That's me*, you are not alone. If enlisting help for yourself doesn't feel worth it, think about this: Stress during pregnancy doesn't just impact you. High cortisol levels, which rise because you are stressed out, can lead to complications and impact your baby's development.

For these reasons and so many others, therapy should be a standard part of pre- and postnatal care. Making time to see a therapist may not feel like it fits into your busy life. But good news: They are available by phone, video chat, and even text message. If that feels like too much, try an app or meditation.

> *Eating my feelings during the miscarriage didn't work very well when it came to pregnancy number two. And by the time we hit number three, I knew I had to work through the past two before I could relax. I've used therapy several times to get through life transitions, so it felt like a natural solution. A friend supplied a referral, and I committed to go as many times as it took to work through my unresolved feelings.*
>
> *Therapy didn't replace my relationships with friends or with Nick. Even with incredible support and love there were still things I just couldn't say out loud to them. And that's the beautiful thing about therapy—you can say anything and the therapist not only won't tell anyone, they actually can't. Legally! For me, therapy is a safe place to unload those secret, sometimes irrational thoughts in a judgment-free environment, and to someone trained to help you make sense of it all.*

### Bodyworkers and massage

Massage is the most common complementary therapy recommended during pregnancy, and for good reason. Massage decreases depression, anxiety, and pain, and can even result in fewer prenatal complications. Women who experience depression during pregnancy may benefit the most from massage, as the rates of prematurity and low birth weight drop along with their cortisol levels.[11]

Outside of helping you feel pampered during pregnancy, massage has big benefits during labor, too. Women who received massage therapy reported labors that were three hours shorter on average, and less need for medication.

Before you run out and book a massage, there are a few things to know. Many therapists will not do it in the first trimester due to a fear of stimulating labor-inducing acupressure points, a worry that is not actually grounded in science. That said, if you're on the conservative side you may want to wait for the full-body rubdown until you are further along.

When booking a massage, no matter how early you are, let your therapist know you are pregnant. They won't tell your whole social circle, and it's really important for them to be able to customize your treatment based on how many weeks into pregnancy you are.

### *Telemedicine*

The idea of communicating medical information at a distance started around 500 BCE in Greece and Rome.[12] Fires, drums, horns, and smoke signals were used to share news about births and deaths, or to signal plague outbreaks. The invention of the telegraph and phone ushered in the modern age of telemedicine, with the launch of services like 911 in 1968. This simple number provided faster and more consistent access to emergency care, and removed the additional time it took for an operator to forward their call to the right place.

Think of today's telemedicine as magical, on-demand access to a wealth of experts through your phone or computer from wherever you happen to be. The types of services available range from primary care appointments to second opinions from specialists, and encompasses every possible expert related to pregnancy and family needs. Convenience factor aside, it allows you to experience much of the above more affordably, without taking time off from work or play, arranging transportation, or hiring a sitter.

Telemedicine is a great resource for pregnancy, but is perhaps even more valuable when you have a wee babe at home. So familiarize yourself with a few services now, kick-test one or two, and then make sure you bookmark the ones that allow you to access pediatricians for late-night questions and those early days when it feels impossible to leave the house.

### *Pelvic floor therapists*

*Kegels, Kegels, Kegels* is the refrain you are likeliest to hear when it comes to strengthening your pelvic floor during pregnancy. But turns out, one in three women can't do them correctly without instruction.[13]

We'll dive more deeply into what the pelvic floor is and how it works in the second trimester. But here's a sneak peek: Your pelvic floor consists of the muscles that support your bladder, your bowel, and—most relevant here—your uterus. Training during pregnancy makes you less likely to experience leaking and incontinence postpartum[14] and can even shorten labor.[15]

In France, *la rééducation périnéale*, or pelvic floor rehabilitation, is a standard part of the postpartum experience. Here in the US, not so much. But more and more research shows that seeing a pelvic floor therapist preventively during pregnancy and postpartum has huge benefits. If you see one early in your pregnancy, they will assess the current state of your pelvic floor and teach you a series of exercises to do at home. Toward the end of the third trimester, you can see them more frequently for treatments like perineal massage, which can help prevent tearing during birth. Afterward, they can help with recovery and conditions like diastasis recti and help you return to an active sex life.

Pelvic floor therapy is generally covered by insurance, so if your practitioner is in network, expect either a copay or reimbursement later.

### *Getting the most out of your care team*

Deciding which providers and practices fit best into your life and align with your values is up to you. Once you assemble your dream team, ensure that you are communicating and making decisions together, and that you share anything important from other appointments.

Another consideration is how you best process information, and what type and amount of data helps you feel confident. For example, if you like to outsource to the experts, you may not care as much about stats and the reasoning behind a care plan. The opposite is true if you are a data-driven person who enjoys analyzing every possible option. No matter where you are on the spectrum, let your providers know so they can calibrate the amount and type of information they provide at appointments.

It's your right to ask as many questions as it takes to feel comfortable—no matter how silly they might seem at the time. This can feel awkward if an appointment feels rushed. Pro tip: Keep a list of questions that come up at home on your phone so you can avoid getting into the car after an appointment and thinking, *I wish I would have asked [fill in blank].*

# MAKING A BABY

Eggs, ovulation, sex, and taking *the* test

Though it probably seems like some couples just look at each other and *bam!* are pregnant, that is not the case for most. You may already know the basics of when and how you can get pregnant from middle school sex ed, your parents, friends, or favorite fertility app. But no matter what you think you know, there are ways to save time and it's important to calibrate your expectations.

*I know what you're thinking: you* are *one of those people who got pregnant every time you tried. Yes, but our fertility hit rate is pretty unusual. However, it was no accident. I followed all the advice below: I learned to understand the ebbs and flows of my cycle, tracked ovulation with a kit, and had sex on the optimal days. I also had weekly acupuncture appointments, which at minimum helped me relax and deal with the ups and downs.*

## THE TRUTH ABOUT YOUR AGE

Fact: The day you turn thirty-five, your eggs do not shrivel up, nor do your odds of getting pregnant go to zero. In fact, there is a dramatic rise in the number of women who wait to have their first child. Since the 1970s, the number of first-time births to mothers thirty-five or older has increased ninefold.[1] The practice of defining "advanced maternal age" as thirty-five or older is more than three decades old, and, just like the term itself, is long overdue for an update.

Here's the truth. You are born with between one and two million eggs. By your first period, your supply has dropped to three hundred thousand. Though you'll ovulate only about four hundred times in your life, each month you'll lose about a thousand potential eggs. But the number of eggs you have does not dictate your ability to get pregnant. In fact, low ovarian reserves are not a good indicator of your overall fertility.[2]

What is true after thirty-five is that egg quality goes down, and your odds of having an embryo with a chromosomal abnormality increase. This is the main cause of higher miscarriage rates and of the rising chance that your child will have a condition like Down syndrome.

During your fertile early twenties, 90 percent of all eggs are normal,[3] and couples have a 96 percent chance of conceiving in under a year. From your fertile peak between twenty-four and thirty-four, your odds go to 86 percent after a year. At thirty, your conception success rate is still high—78 percent through age thirty-nine. At forty, fertility gets a little more complicated. Your odds of getting pregnant each month drop to 5 percent.[4] It's still possible to have a healthy pregnancy, but you might require assistance.

One in 100 women are affected by premature ovarian failure (loss of normal ovarian function) before age forty. If you have a family history, talk to your doctor.

## HOW OVULATION WORKS

It's been a while since you got "the talk" after your first period, so here's a refresher. A typical menstrual cycle is twenty-eight days. Its purpose: to prepare your body for pregnancy. At the beginning of each cycle, estrogen and progesterone mature an egg in one of your ovaries, and make the lining of your uterus thick and spongy. Halfway through your cycle, your right or left ovary (usually they alternate months) releases this mature egg through one of your fallopian tubes into the uterus in a process called ovulation. If the egg is fertilized by sperm, it burrows into the newly thick and inviting uterine lining and begins a pregnancy. If it isn't fertilized, the lining breaks down and the resulting blood and tissue flow out as your period.

For purposes of getting pregnant, your focus is the fertile window before the middle of the cycle—three days before and up to the day of ovulation. It is the most likely time you will successfully become pregnant, as the egg is available to be fertilized for only twelve to twenty-four hours. Sperm, on the other hand, can hang out and live in the reproductive organs for as long as three to five days, which is why having sex *before* you actually ovulate is a more successful route.

So how do you know if you're ovulating? Since every woman's cycle is slightly different, you have to pay attention. There are tried-and-true technology-free methods.[5] And if you want to take things to the next level, you can pair them with one of the many apps and devices available to help you to see trends and, given time, even predict when you'll ovulate based on your cycle's history. Let's look at a few.

### *Cervical mucus method*

Cervical mucus is exactly what it sounds like—mucus that comes out of your cervix as vaginal discharge.

The same hormones that control the menstrual cycle—progesterone and estrogen—also influence the texture and appearance of cervical mucus. Right after your period, it will be light or possibly absent. As the egg matures, mucus increases in the vagina and will gradually get less cloudy. Cervical mucus around ovulation is clear and slippery, sometimes even stretchy, and resembles egg white. This consistency is your sign that ovulation is under way.

If you want to give this method a whirl, get into a comfortable position, and reach one clean finger (index or middle is best) into your vagina and up toward your cervix to take a sample. Look at it and feel the consistency. If there isn't much going on or the mucus is sticky or creamy, it's not quite time. If it's slightly stretchy or wet, ovulation is near. If you get the holy grail of cervical mucus, stretchy egg whites, grab your partner—it's baby-making time. You can also check your underwear or toilet paper if you are in a rush. However, it may be harder to correctly assess what is going on.

Tip: Though many practitioners and women swear by it, this method is not always reliable or easy. It's especially difficult for those with sexually transmitted diseases, bacterial vaginosis or yeast infections, PCOS, previous cervical surgeries, and for users of feminine hygiene products. Cervical mucus monitoring also requires daily monitoring during the times you think you may be fertile.

### Basal body temperature method

This method demands the same daily diligence as cervical mucus monitoring. Your basal body temperature (BBT) is the temperature of your body at rest. To put together an accurate BBT chart, you'll need to take and record your temperature every morning as soon as you wake up, before you get out of bed. No bathroom breaks; you have to do it before you stand up. All you need is a basal body thermometer, which can be found at any drugstore for $10. They take slightly longer to give a result than the instant fever-detecting variety, as an accurate reading to the tenth of a degree makes all the difference.

So what do BBT readings tell you, exactly? During ovulation, your basal body temperature rises slightly from its normal state, by between 0.4 and 0.8°F. The reading won't tell you precisely when the egg is released, but almost all women will ovulate within three days of that spike. BBT will stay at that spiked level until your period starts, then drop down again until the next cycle begins.

Tip: Many people also swear by BBT charting, but factors like sleep quality, having a fever, drinking or smoking the night before, or even going to the bathroom before measuring can throw off its accuracy. BBT needs to be measured at the same time every day to be truly correct.

### The pee-on-a-stick method

Ovulation predictor kits (OPKs) detect the surge in luteinizing hormone (LH) twelve to thirty-six hours before you ovulate. This surge can last just hours, or as long as one to two days. Though there are tests that can be done with saliva or sweat, the most popular fluid input is urine. OPKs can be low-tech color-changing paper strips, or more advanced digital readers with smiley faces and pop-out test sticks, or even fertility monitors that you use all month long.

Each brand has slightly different requirements, so check the directions. The best practice is to test with first-thing-in-the-morning pee, and then again in the afternoon. Drinking too many fluids will dilute the results, so go easy on the liquids before you test.

Tip: Ovulation tests detect only the signs you are *about to* ovulate, but they can't confirm that you actually did. Women with irregular cycles or other menstrual issues like PCOS may have difficulty knowing if and when they ovulate. If you don't get a positive result, it could mean one of several things. If you have a long cycle, you could be testing too soon. If you tested only in the morning, your LH surge might be short and not detectable until the afternoon. You also may not have ovulated that cycle, or could be using a faulty test. This can happen with any brand, but is more common with cheap, bulk-packaged strips.

If you want to know with certainty, consider OPKs training wheels while you're learning the ropes of cervical mucus or BBT monitoring. OPKs are a great complement and when used with another method can paint a more complete picture.

### Fertility sensors

Into the high-tech life? There are an increasing number of sensors and devices designed to make fertility tracking more frictionless, by tracking physiological data and syncing it automagically with an app. Using parameters like skin temperature, resting pulse, heart rate variability, and sleep, they create a score that provides insight into your cycle and other indicators that can help you conceive.

These sensors come in varied form factors, from connected basal body thermometers to a vaginal sensor that measures your core body temperature, and bracelets that track multiple parameters like resting pulse rate, stress, perfusion, and movement while you sleep.

Tip: Before dropping the $100 to $300 they typically cost, check the device's clinical trial data, usually available on its website. Also be sure that your health profile fits the device's patient criteria, as many devices do not work well with fertility-related health conditions.

> *I tried all of these methods and leaned most heavily on OPKs and an app that predicted my ovulation date. Cervical mucus monitoring was not for me, as I had a hard time discerning the different consistencies. And even after leaving a thermometer on my bedside table, inevitably I'd forget and get up to use the loo before using it.*

## DOING IT

Sex while trying to conceive isn't always *Kama Sutra*–level romantic, especially if you've been at it awhile or are attempting to time it with an ovulation peak. If you're not careful, it can start to feel like a job.

So in the spirit of keeping it as stress-free as possible, here are the answers to the most common sex-during-conception questions.

### How many times do we need to do it?

More is not always better. When men ejaculate too frequently, sperm quality and quantity goes down. When it doesn't happen enough, sperm can be too old and slow to get to the egg in a timely fashion. So though it seems logical to have sex five times per day during your fertile window, that is not the best way to get pregnant.

To optimize for sperm quality and getting them to their destination on time, have sex every other day or once per day *at most* in the five days leading up to ovulation and on the day of.

### What are the best positions?

Clinical research into pregnancy-friendly sexual positions is pretty much nonexistent, and no one position has ever been proven more effective than others. But there is a powerful force that you should consider when trying to conceive: gravity. The closer the sperm starts to the cervix, the more likely it is to get where it needs to go.

For that reason, the two most recommended positions are missionary and doggy style. They allow for deep penetration, and in the case of missionary, the sperm is deposited directly into the top of the vagina closer to the cervix. There are many variations, like putting a pillow under your lower back in missionary to tilt your hips up, or lowering down flat from all fours in doggy style. Rather than obsess about form and technique, mix things up and have fun.

### Will staying on my back afterward help?

The meeting of sperm and egg actually happens quickly. The entrance to the uterine canal is only a few centimeters long, and in simulated studies,[6] strong sperm can travel at a rate of five millimeters per minute, completing the whole journey from ejaculation to egg in about ten minutes. They encounter a few barriers along the way in, like cervical mucus that filters out low-quality swimmers. Once the strong sperm make it through the first round of the vaginal obstacle course into the uterus, muscular contractions can help speed things up.

Though there is no hard proof that it makes a difference, not getting up immediately after sex doesn't hurt, and could help. For that reason, some doctors recommend staying on your back with your hips tilted up for ten to twenty minutes to ensure that any sperm that could make it to an egg get their best shot.

Don't be concerned about any fluids that leak out afterward. Less than 5 percent of ejaculate actually contains sperm.

### Anything else that can help my odds?

Avoid douching after sex, and choose your lubricants wisely. If you need a little extra help, make sure your tube doesn't contain spermicide or glycerin, which impedes and kills sperm. Water-based and pH balanced are two lubricant features to seek out, or there are specific products made especially for conception. Don't raise your core body temperature afterward with saunas, hot baths, or intense exercise, either, as those are all sperm-killers.

The don't-make-it-a-job advice isn't just so you and your partner continue to have fun together. Too much stress can lower your chance of getting pregnant, so find ways to relax, and try not to obsess.

## THE WAIT, OR (WHAT FEELS LIKE) THE LONGEST TWO WEEKS OF YOUR LIFE

You've done the deed, you're hoping for the best, and now you have to wait the fourteen or so days before your missed period. Rather than looking for early pregnancy symptoms before that missed period, for your own sanity seek out distractions and try not to think about it too much. As mentioned a hundred times previously, worrying and stress are fertility killers, so do your best to focus your mind on other things.

### *Early signs you might be pregnant*

The most obvious is a missed period. But if you're on the lookout before that happens, there are other signs. You'll notice a lot of these symptoms could be mistaken for PMS. It can be tricky to know the difference, so rather than reading into every single small change, focus on taking good care of yourself until that missed period actually happens.

- Sensitive nipples
- Cramping
- Fatigue
- Nausea
- Frequent peeing (especially at night)
- Change in tastes and smells
- Moodiness
- Implantation bleeding

Implantation bleeding is especially confusing. It may seem counterintuitive, but as many as one-third of women experience spotting around the time the embryo implants in the uterine lining. Here are a few ways to differentiate implantation bleeding from your period:

- **Timing:** Typically happens a few days before your period is due, around ten days after you ovulated
- **Duration:** It can last for just hours or one to two days
- **Color:** Lighter pink or brownish in color versus the more vibrant cranberry color that marks your period
- **Cramping:** More mild cramping than your period, and no growing intensity

## TAKING THE TEST

There are many types of pregnancy tests—digital, strips, composta-
ble, those that involve smiley faces, paper, plastic—the list goes on.
Though you may want to trust only the top-shelf tests with features
like digital readout, the underlying technology for detecting human
chorionic gonadotropin (HCG), the hormone placental cells produced during pregnancy, is the same whether it involves a paper
strip dipped in a cup or a fancy plastic stick you pee on. You'll later
blame HCG for your morning sickness, but for now, its presence in
your urine is the most easily detectable early indicator that you are
indeed pregnant.

With the proliferation of early detection tests claiming the ability
to reveal pregnancy as soon as a week before you miss your period,
it's tempting to pull one out the second it is possible to get a positive.
However, because HCG levels are low early on, you may get a false
negative depending on what time of day you take it and the cycle day.
It's highly unlikely you'll receive a false positive unless you are going
through fertility treatments, as HCG is rarely produced in detectable
levels in the body for any other reason. So even if color on the strip is
on the faint side, you are likely pregnant.

Putting false negatives aside, there is another reason to wait to test.
Chemical pregnancies, or very early miscarriages that happen before
five weeks, are thought to occur in 50 to 60 percent of all first-time
pregnancies,[7] and show the same HCG surge. While they can be
caused by low hormone levels, inadequate uterine lining, or an infection, most commonly they are tied to chromosomal issues. Since
the symptoms of a chemical pregnancy are so much like PMS, most
women never even know they were pregnant.

### When to take the test:

- Though it's *really, really* hard, try to wait until
  your period is due to avoid false negatives and

disappointment. If your period is inconsistent, take your first test at least nineteen days after you tried to conceive.

- Always take a pregnancy test first thing in the morning, since HCG levels are at their most concentrated before your urine is diluted with coffee or other fluids. For the same reason, don't drink ten glasses of water and then test. If you're testing after five weeks, HCG levels should be high enough to get an accurate result any time of day.

### Other seemingly obvious tips:

- Read (and follow) the directions on the test you buy. They can be (and often are) confusing. Even though it all seems intuitive (how hard can it be to hold a stick in a stream of urine?), there are actually ways to do it wrong.
- Check the expiration date (the tests do become less effective over time).

If you want to confirm the test results, make an appointment with your practitioner and request a blood test. You are subject to the same timelines here, as in most cases blood tests require higher HCG levels than urine, which may give you a false negative.

# IF THINGS GET BUMPY

## Understanding fertility issues—
## and what to do if you run into them

**I**f you're here because something has gone wrong, you are in the company of millions who have been there and have gone on to build their families. The ongoing leaps in reproductive technology are staggering—there are more options today than ever before.

If you're nervous to read this section because thinking about what could go wrong scares you, take a deep breath. Talking about miscarriage and fertility challenges more openly is the best way to remove the shame and secrecy surrounding them.

*I'll start by sharing mine. After one cycle to let my decades on the pill settle out, we decided to give conception a shot, assuming it was just a practice round. A few days before my period was due, I woke up feeling like I had the flu. Thinking it couldn't possibly be positive, I decided to take an early detection pregnancy test anyway.*

*And there they were: two pink lines.*

*We never expected to get pregnant so quickly, and were*

*set to go skiing in a remote part of British Columbia. Though strenuous physical activity was no longer in the cards considering my dearth of energy, I still wanted to go and enjoy the scenery. So the small town of Nelson, BC, is where I miscarried.*

*When you know you are pregnant and see blood, it is terrifying. Far from home, I used Maven, a telemedicine platform, to speak with a nurse practitioner, as I had no clue what to do. She advised me to go to the hospital just to make sure everything was okay.*

*An ultrasound and cervix check in the Canadian ER later, doctors took the first of two blood draws to see if my HCG levels were going up or down. Down meant miscarriage, up meant still pregnant. Based on the amount of bleeding, I knew it was likely bad news, but the twenty-four-hour wait to confirm was still excruciating.*

*Unsurprisingly, my HCG levels crashed at the follow-up. It was a miscarriage.*

*Luckily, my body returned to normal without the need for any medical intervention. Emotionally, it was a different story. I knew logically that the miscarriage wasn't my fault. But there is nothing logical about loss. I felt like a total failure, and my mind repeated a chorus of what I should have done differently—started a family years earlier, rested more, stopped drinking any alcohol or caffeine while trying to get pregnant. . . . The self-blame was endless.*

*I knew a few friends had experienced miscarriages, but after I shared what had happened, several more confided that they too had had one, or even more than one. Miscarriage truly is a secret club that no one wants to join, with a members list miles long.*

## MISCARRIAGE

Miscarriage is known by many names: *early pregnancy loss, fetal demise,* and *spontaneous abortion* among them. After twenty weeks, it's called stillbirth. No matter when it happens, miscarriage can be devastating.

Because so many happen before a woman ever knows she's pregnant, and not all are reported, it's nearly impossible to quantify what percentage of pregnancies end in miscarriage. Our best guess is that it happens in 10 to 20 percent of all pregnancies, but it could be as high as one in three.[1] More than a million American women report a miscarriage each year, and 80 percent of these happen in the first trimester.[2] As many as 75 percent happen because of chromosomal problems, errors that occur randomly as the embryo divides, not issues inherited from either parent. Chromosomal issues are more common with age, so the risk of miscarriage goes up when women hit thirty-five, and when men are over forty.

Miscarriage is one of the least talked about bits of the pregnancy process, so myths, misconceptions, and questions abound. It's time to clear them up.

### Myth: It's my fault.

**Fact:** Though it's very hard not to feel this way, miscarriage is rarely "your fault." The majority are caused by chromosomal abnormalities—not by something you ate, stress from your job or partner, or by your working out too hard. Miscarriages can happen no matter how healthy and diligent you are, because the embryo is simply not viable.

We don't really understand why chromosomal abnormalities lead to miscarriage. One theory is that when the mother's immune system detects a problem with the embryo, it is programmed to end the pregnancy. Another is that a genetic problem, missing or extra copies of genes, causes the fetus to stop growing or to grow improperly. Most of these problems happen completely randomly, so unless one or both parents have an underlying genetic issue, they are unlikely to happen again in future pregnancies.

Outside of chromosomal problems, known miscarriage causes are related to uncontrolled health conditions like diabetes, hormonal and thyroid issues, infections, or uterine or cervical abnormalities. The lifestyle-related factors that you can control are being over-weight or underweight, smoking, using drugs, and aggressive alcohol consumption. If you're wondering how to define aggressive alcohol consumption, miscarriage risk increases 6 percent for each drink you have over five per week.[3]

### Myth: If I have one miscarriage, I'm just going to keep having them.

Fact: If you have one miscarriage, it does not mean you will have another one. Fewer than 5 percent of women have two consecutive miscarriages, and only 1 percent experience three or more.[4] Recurrent pregnancy loss is poorly understood but, as the stats indicate, is relatively rare.

If you are concerned, make an appointment with your physician to talk about why your miscarriage might have happened. It's also a good time to consider making any lifestyle adjustments that can improve your overall health. But remember, most miscarriages happen due to chromosomal abnormalities, not something you did wrong, and there was likely nothing you could have done to prevent it.

### How can I tell if I'm having a miscarriage?

Bleeding, especially around the time of implantation, is pretty common, making it hard to know the difference between that and a miscarriage. If you experience bleeding and any of the below miscarriage symptoms, it's time to call your physician:

- Severe abdominal pain
- Cramps
- Progression of vaginal bleeding from light to heavy
- Discharge of tissue with clots
- Fever
- Back pain
- Unexplained weakness

### What do I do if I'm having a miscarriage?

Call your provider. They will ask for the start date of your last period to understand how far along you are, as well as symptoms and any history of fertility issues. Pending your circumstances, they may suggest waiting to see if it resolves, ask you to come into the office, or direct you to a nearby emergency room to get checked out.

If you do go in, a doctor or nurse will do a pelvic exam to see if your cervix is dilated, and an ultrasound to check for a fetal heartbeat and other developmental indications. If it looks like a miscarriage is occurring, a sequence of two blood tests set twenty-four hours apart to see if HCG levels are going up or down is one way they can confirm. If you are passing tissue, that may also be sent to a lab for analysis.

If it's not a miscarriage, your doctor will monitor you until symptoms subside, and suggest you take it easy and minimize any unnecessary travel.

If it is a miscarriage, there are several ways it can resolve. The first is known as *expectant management*, which means letting it take a natural course. A first-trimester miscarriage usually feels and looks like a period. Heavy bleeding or passage of tissue should stop in a few hours, and light bleeding will conclude after several days.

If the miscarriage doesn't or can't clear on its own and it's before nine weeks, your doctor will suggest medication to help things along. It's taken orally or vaginally, and typically works over a twenty-four-hour period. The medications cause bleeding and cramping, and in some cases nausea, vomiting, fever, chills, diarrhea, and headaches. While you likely won't need bed rest, be prepared to take it easy for a few days, and have high-absorbency pads on hand, especially overnight.

If you are nine weeks or more into your pregnancy, you may need a dilation and curettage (D&C) to remove any remaining tissue. This minor surgical procedure can be done in an office, or as a minor out-patient procedure. It takes under thirty minutes and does not require a long recovery period. Your doctor may start the process of dilating your cervix a few hours or the day before the procedure with medica-tion. After it's dilated, the remaining tissue will be removed from your uterus with a long instrument called a curette. You'll spend an hour or two in recovery to check for bleeding or other complications, and for the effects of anesthesia to wear off before you leave. Your blood type checked to make sure you don't need a shot of RhoGAM if your blood type is Rh-negative.

Complications from a D&C are rare, but expect to feel drowsy and have mild cramping and light bleeding. Sex is off-limits for one to two weeks afterward to reduce your infection odds. Your uterus has to build a brand-new lining after a D&C, so your period can take longer than one cycle to come back.

### When can I try to get pregnant again?

Opinions range from as soon as you are medically cleared to have sex again to six months. Exactly how many cycles you should wait generally depends how far along you were when the miscarriage hap-pened, how it resolved, and your overall health.

Most doctors suggest waiting two to three months to let your uterus go back to normal and, if the miscarriage required intervention or your pregnancy was more advanced, monitoring your hormone levels. It's also best to let your cycle get back to its regularly scheduled program.

If it happened early and did not require any medical interven-tion, there is no evidence that shows that waiting even one month contributes to the health of future pregnancies. Ovulation can happen as soon as two weeks after a miscarriage, which means you can get pregnant before your period arrives.

While there is no official consensus on the body, there is on the mind. Most health professionals will tell you that letting yourself heal physically is only half the process, and you should not feel pressured to get pregnant again until you feel ready. Some women are raring to go immediately, and others need time to deal with what happened.

## *Healing after a miscarriage*

There is no right or wrong way to deal with the aftermath of a miscarriage. Whether you choose to lean on friends and family, work with a therapist, or process the experience privately with your partner, the only strategy to avoid is doing it alone. People may not know what to say or do, so be as open as you can and tell them what you need. You may be surprised to find out how many of your friends and family have gone through it, too.

The grief can be much deeper for you, as the pregnancy and loss happened in your body. Because it wasn't as real to them in that way, your partner might process it differently. Try not to judge if they don't seem to feel it as intensely.

Seeing a therapist or counselor who specializes in processing grief or trauma can also be helpful. If you are short on time or money, telemedicine is a more flexible, affordable option.

There are also support groups that allow you to connect with others who have gone through the same loss. Whether you do it in person or online, hearing and reading other people's experiences can be healing, but it can also trigger feelings of grief, so try to manage your consumption if it's causing heartache.

Every single pregnancy is different. You are not doomed to repeat the same thing over and over. Though at first it's hard not to look for bad news every time you're in the bathroom, find distractions and stay engaged with the rest of your life. Meeting friends for dinner, putting time in with a favorite hobby, getting exercise, and even focusing on work can help minimize anxiety as your journey continues.

> *I developed a silly but effective tactic to deal with my doom-and-gloom googling. Every time I reached for my phone to look up a new possible symptom, instead of opening the browser I played a very silly game. Doing that until the urge was forgotten, which didn't take long, was my best coping mechanism.*

## DEALING WITH FERTILITY CHALLENGES

Though, like miscarriage, it still lives largely in the shadows, infertility affects 15 percent of couples.[5] It is now recognized as a disease by leading health organizations around the world; the designation should improve the spotty insurance coverage for fertility treatments.

If you don't fall pregnant right away, remember it's typically a three-to-six-month process. If you're under thirty-five, a year of unprotected sex that does not end in pregnancy is the general guideline before seeking professional help. If you're over thirty-five, you should talk to someone once you hit that six-month mark.

While women are nearly always treated first, 40 to 50 percent of all fertility issues are due to "male factor" infertility[6] and affect 7 percent of all men. In fact, multiple studies show that sperm concentration across North America, Australia, and Europe has declined over 50 percent in the past forty years.[7] Lifestyle factors like stress, obesity, and smoking all reduce sperm count, but scientists believe the growing number of chemical compounds we ingest—especially estrogen and testosterone—could also be culprits.[8]

Men's most common fertility problem is related to sperm: either a low count or poor quality. Sometimes it's caused by lifestyle or past medical issues, but frustratingly, often there is no obvious cause. Women's fertility issues are more varied and can be triggered by everything from PCOS to endometriosis, low ovarian reserves, or a failure to ovulate. The good news is that science has come a long way in diagnosing and treating all of these conditions.

If you encounter challenges, expect your physician to refer you to a reproductive endocrinologist (REI), a medical professional who deals specifically with fertility challenges. At your first appointment, they will talk about your medical history and lifestyle, and run a few tests. Their questions and recommendations will be related to things like whether you are having regular periods, eating well, are over- or underweight, exercising, smoking or using recreational drugs, and ensuring none of your medications interfere with your fertility.

When it comes to tests, here are the initial candidates:

- Everyone's favorite—the Pap smear
- A blood test during your period to check for hormone imbalances, especially FSH, LH, and estradiol
- A blood test to confirm you are actually ovulating during your fertile window
- A urine test for chlamydia (its presence can block your fallopian tubes)

If your partner gets tested, they will also get a urine test for chlamydia, which affects sperm function, and a check for abnormal sperm shapes or poor motility. Pending the results of the sperm analysis, they may also undergo further blood tests, a testicular biopsy, or a karyotype to determine if there are any chromosomal abnormalities.

If the results are inconclusive after your first visit, your REI will run further diagnostics. These include:

- A full hormone panel to measure any other imbalances
- An ultrasound to take a look at your uterus and ovaries
- A series of ultrasound scans to see if an egg is developing over time
- A hysterosalpingogram, a procedure that uses X-ray imaging to confirm your fallopian tubes are open and working
- A hysteroscopy, aka a procedure that allows your doctor to look inside your uterus with a camera to check for fibroids and polyps

Genetic testing is another option, as there are screens for fertility-related risk factors that allow a more personalized treatment plan.

## BACKUP PLANS

### *IUI*

The first line of defense if things aren't happening, or if you're conceiving with donor sperm, is intrauterine insemination (IUI). IUI closes the time and distance sperm have to travel to the egg by depositing sperm directly into the uterus during ovulation. It is done if you have unexplained infertility, diminished ovarian reserves, PCOS, or an irregular cycle, or if your partner's or donor's sperm are of low motility or quality. Some women need fertility medications to help things along or hormones to trigger ovulation, too. Your partner's or donor's sperm will also be evaluated for health and motility.

When it's ovulation time, a sperm sample goes through a process called washing to ensure only the healthy, motile specimens remain. That sample is then inserted through a thin tube through the cervix and directly into the uterus around the time of ovulation. Insemination takes only five to ten minutes at your doctor's office, or in a fertility clinic, and doesn't require any anesthesia. Some people report cramping, but otherwise the whole process is pretty painless. If the sperm and egg come together, and the fertilized embryo implants in your uterus, you're pregnant.

IUI is the most affordable place to start exploring alternative conception methods, at $300 to $1,000 per session.

## IVF

On July 25, 1978, Louise Brown came into the world at Royal Oldham Hospital in the UK. As the first baby conceived and born via in vitro fertilization (IVF), she paved the way for the more than eight million IVF babies[9] born around the world since.

Due to the expense and the physical and emotional toll the treatments can take, if IUI is an option, fertility clinics will start there. IVF is typically used in women with blocked or damaged fallopian tubes, ovulation disorders, or uterine fibroids; when a woman's partner has decreased sperm count or motility; when one or both partners have a genetic disorder; or if there is unexplained infertility. It can be done with your egg and your partner's sperm, or donor sperm and eggs, and can involve a gestational carrier or surrogate.

Women who have been through IVF often describe it as an emotional and hormonal roller coaster, due to the high costs and uncertainty, not to mention the effects of the daily shots that actually pump you full of hormones. It's also not without risks. IVF increases the likelihood of multiple births, miscarriage odds climb to 15 to 25 percent,[10] and 2 to 5 percent of women have an ectopic pregnancy.

IVF starts with an examination of the ovaries and hormone level checks, and pending results, fertility medications to stimulate egg production are prescribed. After a few weeks, eggs are retrieved through a minor surgical procedure that uses ultrasound imaging to guide a hollow needle through the pelvic cavity. You may feel a little sore or bruised, and have cramps and spotting after the retrieval. At the same time, your partner gives a sample of sperm.

At this point, the work is handled by embryologists, or the lab scientists who actually create embryos for implantation. They start by isolating the sperm from the semen, and the eggs from the ovarian fluid. Then, the egg and sperm are combined, and the resulting fertilized eggs are sent to an incubator to develop. Each embryo is monitored and checked during development, and tested for chromosomal abnormalities. If an embryo makes the grade, three to five days after fertilization it is ready for transfer, or frozen to be used later.

Your fertility clinic will tailor the transfer specifically to your needs, but in general, specialists recommend single embryo transfer to avoid risks associated with multiple births. The transfer itself starts just like a Pap smear, as the physician will use a speculum to gain access to the cervix. A fine tube is passed through the cervix using ultrasound guidance, and the embryos are inserted into the uterus. Outside of the same Pap smear–level discomfort, and a full bladder to help the ultrasound, it's normally pain-free.

If the cycle is successful, implantation occurs six to ten days after an egg retrieval during the dreaded two-week wait.

Your physician may have fertility clinic recommendations, but if you'd like to do your own research, the Society for Assisted Reproductive Technology (SART) includes data on over 90 percent of reproductive clinics and powers the CDC's yearly Assisted Reproductive Technology (ART) report.

IVF is not cheap, and insurance does not always cover it, which is why many couples explore other methods before starting. A single IVF cycle can cost between $10,000 and $17,000.

### Gamete donation

When one or both partners cannot provide their own egg or sperm, usually due to poor quality or the risk of passing down genetic

disorders, gamete donation makes it possible to experience pregnancy and birth and, when possible, allows one partner to maintain
a genetic connection to the baby.

Donor material can be sourced from reproductive centers, donor
agencies and banks, or from family members and friends. Before a
donor is accepted, they go through a health screening that includes
medical history, genetic risks, STDs, and a physical. There are long-
term ramifications of genetic connections, so the screening also
includes a psychological component, and counseling for both the
donor and intended parents is highly recommended. The donor's
motivations can vary widely, especially if it is someone who will be
part of the child's life, so it's best to understand them before moving
forward. As intended parents, you should also think about how—or
if—you would eventually tell your child that they do not share your
genetic makeup.

Legally, an agreement will be put in place outlining everyone's
roles, obligations, and expectations. This includes everything from
financial arrangements to possible future contact, and is especially
important if the donor is someone you know. Parentage laws for the
donor and intended parents vary by state and even county, so clarify
and paper everything with legal counsel if you start down this path.

### Surrogacy and gestational carriers

The number of births that involve a gestational carrier or surrogate has
more than doubled since 2013. The reasons are myriad that a woman
cannot carry a baby to term—life-threatening congenital abnormalities, a nonfunctional or missing uterus (yes, some women are born
without one), conditions like pulmonary hypertension, cancer treatments, or more than five pregnancy losses. Surrogacy and gestational
carriers are also options for LGBTQ couples or single parents.

But first, you may be wondering why anyone would sign up for
the job of carrying someone else's child. The reasons to become a

surrogate or gestational carrier can be financially motivated but are also usually personal, and if you interview a few, you'll find everyone has a different answer. What they share is a love of either all or some part of the pregnancy experience, combined with a desire to help prospective parents achieve their dream of building a family. Many cite family members or friends who experienced fertility issues and, having had an easy delivery themselves, a wish to pay it forward.

How do you decide which is right for you? If you have embryos ready to transfer via IVF, a gestational carrier is your best bet. If your eggs cannot be used, choosing between a surrogate or gestational carrier comes down to deciding where the egg comes from.

A gestational carrier becomes pregnant via IVF, and has a gestational relationship, but no genetic relationship with the embryo. A surrogate traditionally uses her own eggs, fertilized via IUI or IVF with your partner's or a donor's sperm, meaning she has a genetic and gestational relationship.

Candidates should be between the ages of twenty-one and forty, have had at least one uncomplicated pregnancy, no more than three cesarean deliveries and no more than five pregnancies total, and no chronic medical conditions. A psychological screening is also important, especially with surrogates, as there is a genetic link. This means addressing any religious and ethical views that could complicate the handoff of the infant later.

Cost is a big consideration, as both are an average of $90,000 to $130,000 in the US, and only slightly cheaper in other parts of the world. You can find one through agencies, IVF clinics, specialized attorneys, and online. This raises another essential aspect: putting a legally binding contract into place. You and the surrogate or carrier must have your own separate legal representation, then agree to terms regarding the pregnancy and your designation as the legal parents.

If the cost and complication of finding someone puts this option out of reach, family members sometimes volunteer. Consider this carefully before agreeing, as it can be much more emotionally complex than enlisting a stranger. The American Society of Reproductive Medicine's list of guidelines is helpful if you explore this direction.

## *Adoption*

There are more than a hundred thousand children in the US looking for homes, and 153 million orphans worldwide. Adoption is complex and takes time, but is generally more affordable than other options.

In the United States, there are four main types of adoption:

**Public agency adoptions** place infants and children who were removed from their homes. You'd begin as foster parents and if it is not in the child's best interest to be reunited with their biological parents, there is a pathway to permanent adoption. It is not the best option if you would like to adopt an infant, though it is cheaper than agency or independent adoptions.

In a **licensed private agency adoption**, birth parents and adoptive parents work through an agency. Birth parents sign away their parental rights but can be involved with the selection of the adoptive family, and future contact is negotiated. The final consent doesn't happen until after the baby is born, which means the birth parents can change their minds. The costs are high, and can take longer than public agency adoptions.

**Independent adoption** is similar to licensed private agency and just replaces the agency with an attorney. The timeline is hard to predict, and the same laws around consent exist. Costs are highly variable depending on the legal agreement.

**Facilitated** or **unlicensed agency adoption** has little oversight and relies on a facilitator to connect birth parents and adoptive parents. If you choose this route, check with your state's guidelines, as it's not legal everywhere, and there is little recourse if things go sideways.

An international adoption can take anywhere from one to five years, and requires the adopting parents to be US citizens. Every country has slightly different rules, so look into specific eligibility requirements. Costs are typically between $15,000 and $45,000.

The State Department hosts a list of approved service providers. Ask for references or attend informational sessions with providers you are considering before making a commitment. They should also be able to help you put together a dossier that contains eligibility paperwork to get things into process.

## TRIMESTER-ZERO CHECKLIST

- [ ] Start taking prenatal vitamins one to three months before you try to conceive.
- [ ] Clean up your lifestyles.
- [ ] Schedule preconception checkups.
- [ ] Get necessary immunizations if you're not up to date.
- [ ] Check the safety of your prescription medications and compatibility with pregnancy.
- [ ] Quit birth control and get to know your cycle.
- [ ] Check your insurance coverage (or sign up for a plan).
- [ ] Talk about your parenting goals.
- [ ] Schedule an appointment with a return-to-work coach.
- [ ] Try not to make having sex a job.
- [ ] Sleep!

# The First Trimester

**N**ow that you're pregnant—or reading ahead—let's get a few things out of the way.

You probably won't look like a celebrity traipsing breezily across the pages of *People* magazine in a flawless maternity ensemble. You will not wake up every day feeling or looking great. You might experience the joys of morning sickness, back pain, fatigue, and all the rest. Or you might not.

Also important: *You may not like being pregnant.* Many women don't!

But even if you follow what your doctor and every other "expert" recommends to the letter, your pregnancy will not be perfect.

To all you fellow type As out there, if conception didn't already teach you this lesson, now is the time to grow comfortable with the idea that you are not in full control of this process. Pregnancy is great training for parenting because even when you do everything right, *things will not always go the way you expect.* More opinions and data are not always better—sometimes they're just more. And the more you obsess over every micro decision, the crazier you will drive yourself.

> *I learned the stop-micromanaging lesson the hard way. My work exposes me to companies that allow people to manage their health outside a clinical setting. It was through their products that I put my ulcerative colitis (a type of irritable bowel disorder) into remission in my late twenties. After keeping a food and lifestyle diary for a year, I identified my triggers and eliminated them. A decade later, my condition is still under control.*
>
> *So I thought, if I could kick ulcerative colitis into remission, why not use similar methods during pregnancy? At minimum, it would make me feel like I had some sort of say over the mass of crazy happening to my body. And maybe it would help lessen my symptoms.*

*Rookie move. I tried out more than twenty apps and ser-*
*vices, most of which were not very useful. When I finally*
*settled on one, I diligently tracked my symptoms and weight,*
*and the app's other desired inputs daily the first two times I*
*was pregnant. That same app provided updates on the baby's*
*size and development, which I also read almost every day.*
*Unlike managing my IBD, none of it improved my symp-*
*toms at all, and frankly, it stoked some pretty unhealthy ten-*
*dencies. The content brought up all the things that could go*
*wrong, and what should be happening each day (as if all*
*pregnancies are the same!), which made me feel like I was a*
*huge failure when anything deviated from the guidelines.*

*There can be huge differences between pregnancies—even*
*if they are close together and you do exactly the same thing.*
*So when I fell pregnant for the third time, I continued to make*
*healthy choices, but also chose to chill out and try to just listen*
*to my body. And instead of silently worrying, I was open when*
*I struggled or needed to talk. Letting go made the whole experi-*
*ence much more enjoyable.*

*This pregnancy was nothing like the first two. No nau-*
*sea, my fatigue level was a 5 instead of a 9, and I generally*
*felt clearer and more like myself. Now that I was a more*
*functional human, the first trimester whizzed by. We navi-*
*gated the gauntlet of tests and appointments as best we*
*could, though it was still difficult not to be anxious or imag-*
*ine all the things that could go wrong.*

*So, as you head into this brave new world, remember*
*that every pregnancy is different. Every pregnant body is*
*different. Yours will be different if you get pregnant again.*
*Sometimes pregnancy feels like an amazing, magical cruise*
*gliding toward the destination of your dreams, and other*
*times it feels like a hijacking—of your body, your mind, and*
*your freedom.*

## SO WHAT'S HAPPENING IN THERE?

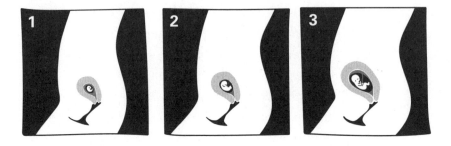

### Month 1

**Baby:** For the first two weeks, your uterus is playing the waiting game until ovulation. Once the egg and sperm meet at the start of week three, they'll start the fertilization process and the resulting cell will begin to divide and implant into the uterine lining in week four. The amniotic and yolk sacs are also forming at the end of the first month, and the brand-new embryo is around the size of a poppy seed.

**You:** Think of month one as bonus month. Most symptoms don't start until around six weeks, but as we've established, every pregnancy (and person) is different. You may have spotting around implantation, which is typically six to twelve days after you conceive. Fatigue, more frequent trips to the restroom, breast tenderness, and morning sickness can show up toward the end of this month, though outside of bloating and fuller breasts, you will probably look the same.

### Month 2

**Baby:** The embryo is growing at a rapid clip—in fact, by the end of the fifth week its heart alone will be the size of a poppy seed. The embryonic period, which spans weeks five to ten, is all about establishing the foundations of the major systems, including the neural tube (the future spinal cord and brain), the circulatory system, the kidneys, the lungs, the mouth, the eyes, and the arm and leg buds. The embryo will close out week eight around the size of that prenatal vitamin you've been taking every day.

**You:** Month two can be a tough one. Symptoms and surging hormones can wreak havoc on your emotions, which may be all over the place now that the reality of pregnancy is setting in. Morning sickness and other digestion-related issues may start along with fatigue, headaches, frequent peeing, and breast changes. No symptoms? Consider yourself lucky, as feeling normal is normal, too. You may start to notice your clothes getting tighter, as your uterus has grown from the size of a fist to that of a roll of toilet paper.

### Month 3

**Baby:** The embryo kicks off this month around the size of the tip of your index finger, and will officially graduate to the rank of fetus in week eleven. Hair follicles, nail beds, bones, cartilage, and muscles are forming, allowing arm and leg movement alongside the beginnings of digestion and hormone production. It is also time for your first prenatal appointment, where you'll hear the heartbeat for the first time. It's an incredible moment—enjoy. By the close of week thirteen, aka the end of the first trimester, the fetus will be about the size of a baseball.

**You:** If you are experiencing the pains of pregnancy symptoms like morning sickness, this month is when they usually peak. Take solace that when you enter the second trimester, you'll start to feel better. Vacillating between irritable, irrational, and joyful is completely normal, as is bursting into tears over cute baby animals. But if you find your downs far outnumber your ups, depression during pregnancy is a symptom to address early. After week ten, morning sickness and aversions can start to diminish, and your appetite may pick up. Your waist will start to get thicker, meaning the days of wearing your prepregnancy pants without getting creative are numbered.

## SYMPTOMS AND SOLUTIONS

While the saying "eating for two" isn't accurate, sleeping for two almost certainly will be. Many women describe the first trimester as the worst trimester for two reasons: You won't actually look pregnant for a while, so nice side effects like strangers giving up subway seats or lifting your bag into the overhead bin are unlikely. And since you probably aren't telling the whole world yet, you will suffer much of this in silence. Hang on—#itgetsbetter.

The severity and prevalence of symptoms are impossible to predict. Some people experience all of them; a lucky few have none. Most are somewhere in the middle. While you're in the throes, just remember: As miserable as they can be, it's all temporary.

### If you have any of these symptoms, call your doctor:

- Vaginal bleeding
- Persistent vomiting
- Blurred vision
- Chills or fever
- Headache that doesn't resolve with water or acetaminophen
- Sudden swelling of hands or face
- Fluid leaking from vagina

*Just because you have morning sickness in one pregnancy does not mean you'll have it in another. My first two pregnancies were nauseous miseries. Like my mom before me, I never actually threw up, but man did I want to. My third was blissfully free of morning sickness, but my reflux was constant, from positive test through birth and even after.*

*Super smell was also a struggle. The hardest moments were enclosed spaces with odorous people and things. Worst of all were car air fresheners. I had to stick my head out the window like a dog just to make it through a rush-hour ride.*

## FOR PARTNERS

Though it will be all about Mom for the next nine months (then all about the baby for eighteen years after that), finding out you're expecting is a huge transitional time for you as well. Your partner doesn't have much control over what's happening in there and might sometimes feel like a different person. The raging hormones, physical transformations, and abundance of unsolicited "advice" she'll receive for the next nine months can really throw her for a loop. She may not always know how or want to ask for help, which is why you have to take more initiative. Here are a few simple ways to get started.

### *Communicate*

Pregnancy brings on brand-new emotions, stress, and occasional (sometimes frequent!) out-of-character behavior. Don't assume you know how she feels or what she needs. Ask, and be prepared to act on whatever she says. Even if she demands something gross, like a chicken-and-banana sandwich.

## First-trimester symptoms and solutions

|  | When does it happen? | Symptoms |
| --- | --- | --- |
| **Morning sickness (aka all-day sickness)** | Typically starts around week 5 or 6, peaks around 9 or 10, then disappears in your second trimester | Nausea, vomiting, aversions to foods and certain smells, cravings |
| **Fatigue** | One of the earliest symptoms that persists in the first and third trimesters and subsides during the second | Falling asleep in the middle of the afternoon, craving a 7 p.m. bedtime, inability to pry yourself out of bed in the morning |
| **Gas and bloating** | Can start immediately or closer to the start of the second trimester | Gas, bloating, feeling like your abdomen is inflated like a bicycle tire |
| **Heartburn and reflux** | Can start immediately or in the second and third trimesters when things start getting more crowded | Burning sensation in your throat or chest, and/or the taste of bile after a meal |
| **Food aversions and cravings** | Can persist throughout pregnancy but lessens in the third trimester | Sensitivity to odors and changing taste preferences |

| Cause | Solutions |
|---|---|
| Caused by rising levels of pregnancy hormones, scientists suspect it evolved to prevent dangerous substances and our varied diets from hurting development, as it occurs primarily when the baby's core organ systems are formed.[1] | Eat small meals and snacks slowly and frequently, drink fluids between meals, and avoid trigger smells. Acupuncture, sipping mint- or citrus-flavored water, enjoying ginger tea or chews, using acupressure bands, and taking a walk can also help. |
| Sky-high progesterone levels | Eat healthy foods (avoid processed and packaged foods), try to get some exercise, take walks and breathe in the fresh air, sleep. |
| Progesterone causes the gastrointestinal tract to relax, slowing down digestion so nutrients can enter the bloodstream and reach your baby. | Eat more fiber, take your time and eat smaller meals, up your water-drinking game. |
| Surging progesterone levels relax the valve between your stomach and esophagus, allowing bile to travel back up. | Eat smaller, more frequent meals; avoid acidic foods like citrus and tomatoes, fatty, oily, fried and spicy foods, and caffeine; do not lie down right after a meal. |
| Hormonal changes | Keep serving sizes small when indulging in unhealthy cravings, or distract yourself if ice cream dreams are all-consuming. If vegetables sound or smell terrible, try blending them into a smoothie with fruit to hide the offensive texture or taste. |

## First-trimester symptoms and solutions (continued)

| | When does it happen? | Symptoms |
|---|---|---|
| **Tender or swollen breasts** | Can be one of the first pregnancy symptoms; acute symptoms typically diminish in a few weeks but will persist on and off throughout pregnancy. | Sore or sensitive breasts and nipples |
| **Acne** | Mostly the first and second trimesters | Teenage-style breakouts that can happen all over your body |
| **Peeing all the damn time** | Another early pregnancy symptom that peaks around weeks 6 to 8. Will lessen by the end of the first trimester, then pick up again in the third with the increased pressure on your bladder. | Needing the loo urgently throughout the day and several (many?) times in the middle of the night |
| **Constipation** | Can be one of the first pregnancy symptoms, will persist throughout pregnancy | Cramping, bloating, farting, gassiness, and inability to poop |
| **Super smell** | Early pregnancy symptom that can persist until birth. | Ability to smell anything from across a room more vividly. Unearthly aversion to cigarette smell. |

| Cause | Solutions |
| --- | --- |
| Hormonal changes | Avoid the shower spray and other unnecessary contact, get fitted for a new bra, or transition into a sports bra. |
| Progesterone. Again. And fluid retention. | Eat well, drink water, and keep your face, body, and hair clean. Do not use spot treatments that contain salicylic acid. |
| Increased blood volume in your body causes kidneys to process extra fluid that goes into your bladder. | Stop drinking liquids a few hours before bedtime. Lean forward when you pee to make sure you're really done. Regulate caffeine intake. |
| Those pesky high-progesterone levels slowing down your digestive system | Drink plenty of fluids, up your fiber intake, and exercise. Mirlax or a generic equivalent is great. Do not take laxatives—they can cause dehydration and uterine contractions. Find ways to relax—stress makes it worse! |
| Estrogen | Carry products scented with citrus (especially lemon) or mint and sniff as needed. Put baking soda in your refrigerator. Make your partner take out the trash. Stay out of enclosed spaces. |

### Remind her she's beautiful and loved

A pregnant body is a miraculous, beautiful thing. That does not mean that all women feel miraculous or beautiful while pregnant, especially in the later stages. Don't be shy about telling her often how much you love her. Share your excitement, and help her overcome self-consciousness related to physical changes.

### Become a pregnancy pro

Though you aren't actually pregnant, you can follow along and mentally prepare for how she will change, the challenges she will face, and when and how her energy will fluctuate. Stepping up especially during the times of greatest change to help around the house or do something kind (foot rubs, date nights, letting her have the run of the Netflix account) can make a world of difference.

### Attend and take notes during doctor's appointments

The idea of a growing baby inside a woman's body is often an abstract concept—until you hear a heartbeat and experience your first ultrasound. Attending doctor's appointments makes everything feel more real, and it's an opportunity for you to pitch in while she's covered in goo or being poked and prodded. Take notes, and make sure you have a record of follow-up or action items. For extra points, keep a note on your phone about questions the two of you have between appointments so nothing slips. Even if your practitioner uses electronic medical records or sends you after-visit notes, you'll be surprised by how much information you immediately forget.

# PREGNANCY FAQ, LIGHTNING ROUND

Bite-size answers to everything you secretly wonder about pregnancy (but are too afraid to ask)

Inevitably, you've started trolling the Internet for answers to pregnancy questions large and small. When you spend enough time in forums (and it really doesn't take long!), you'll run into some kooks. If not, get ready to be pummeled by strangers with anecdotes, uninformed (yet strong) opinions, and bad science.

To protect your sanity, below are the most popular pregnancy questions answered with evidence-based data. They range from things you might be too embarrassed to ask, like does sleeping on your stomach crush the baby (nope!) and can I still have sex (yep!), to topics like how to prevent stretch marks (you can't!) and what are those brown splotches on my cheeks (ack, melasma!)?

### OMG I accidentally had too many cocktails right before I found out I was pregnant! Did I hurt my baby?

You're not alone, especially if you're taking a laissez-faire approach to getting pregnant, or it was unplanned. If your main concern is fetal alcohol syndrome, it is typically associated with heavy drinking during an entire pregnancy, not a onetime event.

A rager before your missed period will likely not cause any lasting or major harm. If it had, it probably would have ended as a miscarriage before you ever knew you were pregnant. If it happened in the first weeks after a missed period, there is more risk, though it's still small. If you are concerned, talk to your doctor.

### What do you mean my doctor won't see me until I'm eight to ten weeks pregnant?!

Yes, it's true—most care providers require that you be at least eight weeks in before your first appointment. Sometimes it's ten. This is for a number of reasons. It's hard to see much on the ultrasound before that time, or do anything other than confirm the pregnancy with a blood test. And since there is nothing a doctor can do to prevent a miscarriage from happening, it's best to wait until things are farther along.

If you have a complicated medical history, are on medications with possible side effects, are otherwise high risk (e.g., diabetes, high blood pressure, seizure disorder), or just really can't wait that long, care providers will often make an exception and see you earlier.

### Do I have to stop baths, steam rooms, hot tubs, saunas, and (gasp) hot yoga while I'm pregnant?

Pregnancy is not the time to take up Bikram. All of these activities cause your core body temperature to increase. When it's too elevated, it causes a condition called hyperthermia, which can be dangerous. The main issue: there are several (admittedly limited) studies that show a connection between neural tube defects and time in hot tubs during the first trimester.[1] Add to that spending time in an enclosed heated space or immersed in hot water makes pregnancy symptoms like dizziness and light-headedness worse.

If you want more detail, here you go: since hot tubs are typically set to 104 degrees, and saunas are sometimes even hotter, it takes only ten to twenty minutes for you to heat up to 102 degrees, which is the magic core body temperature current research suggests avoiding. Your warm nightly bath or morning shower is fine since your entire body isn't covered, but the water temperature shouldn't take an adjustment period; it should be comfortable immediately.

To be safe, avoid anything that would cause you to overheat in the first trimester, and if you must indulge in a steam or sauna in the second or third, keep your visits short.

## How do I figure out my due date?

It's really best to look at it as a due-date *range*, since only about 5 percent of babies arrive when expected. That said, there are a few ways to calculate your estimated due date (EDD). The most common: Add seven days to the first day of your last period, then count nine months forward. Or take the route of less math: your EDD is forty weeks after the first day of your last period. There are also loads of apps that will do the heavy lifting for you if you supply your LMP.

An ultrasound at eleven to fourteen weeks is a less common way your practitioner may choose to date the pregnancy, which can be more precise if ovulation happened on a different cycle day. But don't expect the EDD to change as your pregnancy continues. Even though they will take some measurements during ultrasounds, your practitioner will likely stick with the first-trimester date as it's more accurate.

## Can I have sex while I'm pregnant?

Sure can! Sex will not hurt the baby, and the baby will not see anything requiring therapy later. The better question is what your sex drive will be like. Often it dips in the blah first trimester, comes back raging in the second (increased blood flow down there! More energy!), then goes back down in the third, when the bump gets in the way of pretty much everything. It's best to just pay attention, relax, and go with what feels good at the time.

The exception: if you have a high-risk pregnancy (e.g., placenta previa or shortened cervix) and your care provider cautions against it. Same if you have pain during sex.

### What if I don't have any symptoms, or they stop?

Feel fortunate and enjoy it! If symptoms stop and aren't accompanied by anything else like bleeding or cramping, it doesn't mean you aren't pregnant anymore, or that something is wrong. Morning sickness, discomfort, hormonal surges, and the like come and go. Their absence or presence doesn't predict an empty ultrasound at your next prenatal appointment.

### When can I tell people I'm pregnant?

This is a question with no right answer. Traditionally, most people wait to tell anyone but close friends and family until after the twelve-week mark, when the risk of miscarriage drops and you've heard the heartbeat. Others who've had more complicated journeys may wait until after the twenty-week anatomy scan, when they feel assured everything is okay. Still others can't wait to share with the whole world, and post their first sonograms. If this is you, just be sure that you are equipped to field questions if anything goes wrong.

When it comes to work, if you can wait to tell your boss and coworkers until the second trimester, that's what most people recommend.

### When will I feel the baby moving?

You have a little while before this happens. Most first-time mothers feel movement—also called the quickening—around eighteen to twenty weeks. If this is not your first pregnancy, it can be as soon as thirteen to sixteen weeks. The timing can vary widely, so don't worry if it's not on that exact timeline.

You also may not even realize it's happening, as the first twinges are subtle. They feel like flutters, or even just gas or indigestion. In time you will recognize kicks and punches and be able to detect a distinct pattern and schedule as you move into the third trimester. And toward the end, you'll wish for a break from the rib kicks and middle-of-the-night hiccups.

*Yes, feeling your baby move is absolutely amazing and surreal. Having an actual human being growing inside your body is also really weird to contemplate.*

*I spent the entire third trimester dealing with contraction-causing kicks to the ribs and hiccups every night at 3 a.m. Both were aggressive enough to wake me up and required pacing and jiggling around until they stopped.*

### Why is my skin changing color?

The culprit: skin cells called melanocytes. Their job is to produce melanin, the pigment that causes you to tan in the sun. The surges of estrogen and progesterone during pregnancy cause melanocytes to kick into overdrive and produce more melanin where they are most concentrated, like areas with previous skin damage, your areolas, and the connective tissue that goes down the middle of your stomach. During pregnancy, this brown line bisecting your belly, also known as the linea nigra, becomes more prominent, especially with sun exposure. It fades in the months after birth.

The other common skin issue is melasma, or "the mask of pregnancy." It appears as dark patches on your face, especially the forehead, nose, and cheeks. These skin issues will resolve on their own a few months after birth or when you conclude breastfeeding, so skip the lightening creams and laser treatments.

### Is pregnancy brain real?

Sorry, can you repeat the question?

As pregnancy wears on, your ability to communicate or remember what you had for breakfast can get worse due to declining sleep quality. But here's the real cause of your forgetfulness: Your brain actually shrinks during pregnancy and doesn't return to its original size until two years postpartum.[2] We don't really know why. But the loss of gray matter doesn't mean you are getting dumber. The theory is that the contraction actually makes the brain more efficient in responding to your baby's needs, and increases maternal attachment.

### What's with all the peeing?

The culprit: the hormone HCG, as it increases the blood flow to your kidneys and pelvic area. Frequent peeing starts around the time you miss your period; gets better during the second trimester, when the uterus rises and takes pressure off your bladder; and is even more frequent in the final weeks of the third trimester, when the baby's head drops back on your bladder. Don't avoid water or fluids, as pregnancy puts women at increased risk of UTIs and it's much easier to get dehydrated.

### How do I prevent stretch marks?

Skip the expensive lotions, creams, and brews promising a perfectly smooth postpartum belly. Getting stretch marks or not is largely a function of genetics. If your mom had them during pregnancy, or if you already have a history of stretch marks, you may also get them. Stretch marks also happen when your skin can't keep up with how quickly your body is expanding. So outside of being born with the right genes, gaining weight gradually is your best defense.

Though no amount of cocoa butter or fancy oils can prevent stretch marks entirely, they can help make them less obvious and relieve the itching from your growing bump. Bonus: Slathering on lotion is a nice way to feel pampered, and rubbing it on your legs and ankles can help promote better circulation.

### I don't want to wait until the second trimester to learn the gender! How can I find out now?

Read enough forums and you'll find plenty of ways to "predict" gender early. These include the Ramzi method (based on chromosome polarity—if early ultrasounds show the placenta forming on the right side of your body it's a boy, left it's a girl), how you're carrying (belly it's a boy, hips it's a girl), length of linea nigra (if it stops at your belly button, it's a girl, all the way to your ribs it's a boy), fetal heart rate (over 140 means a girl, under means a boy), and Chinese and Mayan birth tables. Though it can be tempting to try them all, there is no proof that any are accurate. The only potentially plausible gender detection trick is the presence of morning sickness, as female fetuses are associated with higher HCG levels, aka the trigger for nausea.[3]

The earliest way to definitively learn gender is the noninvasive prenatal testing (NIPT) at ten weeks. Chorionic villus sampling (CVS) can also provide answers at ten to thirteen weeks, amniocentesis at fifteen to twenty weeks, or if you wait until your anatomy ultrasound at eighteen to twenty-two weeks, the genitalia are developed enough to be visible. There are risks with CVS and amnio, so if you don't otherwise need those tests and opt out of NIPT, be patient and wait until the anatomy scan. If you are over thirty-five or have other risk factors, your doctor will order an NIPT automatically anyway.

*I put the gender-prediction theories to the test. The results were mixed. My linea nigra to the ribs, carrying in the belly, and no nausea said boy (correct!); Chinese birth table and Ramzi said girl (incorrect!); fetal heart rate differed between appointments, and hence was inconclusive.*

## Will sleeping on my stomach squash the baby?

No. Stomach sleeping will become very uncomfortable as your pregnancy wears on, but the amniotic sac provides plenty of cushion so your baby doesn't turn into a pancake.

*Trust me—you won't even want to sleep on your stomach. What you will want is one of those extremely unsexy wraparound body pillows so you and your bump can get some rest. I wanted to torch mine by the end (my water broke all over it, so instead of ritual burning it just went in the trash), but it was a lifesaver in getting sleep from the middle of the second trimester to birth.*

## Will lying on my back hurt the baby?

No, there is no proof that you will harm the baby if you lie on your back. However, it will probably make you dizzy and want to turn over. The added weight of the baby and their home and accessories compresses the vein that carries blood from the lower half of your body up the right side to your heart. For this reason, many women prefer their left side starting at around twenty weeks, as lying on the right sometimes has a similar effect.

## Will my nose spread and feet grow an extra size?

Feet can grow and spread during pregnancy and stay that way, thanks to the extra weight you cart around for almost a year, and to the effects of the hormone relaxin. And yes, your nose can grow, too, courtesy of the increased, estrogen-related blood flow to your mucous membranes, with more rhinitis and postnasal drip as well. Luckily, that one is temporary and your nose will revert back to its original size after you give birth. Another surprise change later: an expanded rib cage, also caused by relaxin.

### Why shouldn't I change my cat's litter box?

While it's more connected with eating uncooked and cured meats, the issue is an infection called toxoplasmosis, which can be passed through your purring ball of love's feces to your growing baby. It's uncommon in full-grown indoor cats, but if you have three or more kittens while you are pregnant, your odds of infection increase.[4] It's unlikely to be an issue, but hey, pregnancy is a great excuse to hand off poop-scooping responsibilities.

### Wait, I shouldn't garden either?

A more likely source of toxoplasmosis than emptying the kitty litter is working with soil.[5] Interestingly, it also involves our feline friends. If your flower beds are a haven for the bathroom activities of neighborhood cats, the parasites excreted by those infected with toxoplasmosis can live for up to a year in the water or dirt. So if your nesting instinct inspired you to plant a vegetable garden, wear gloves, and be sure to wash everything that comes out of it thoroughly. Same goes for produce in general—if it grows in the ground, give it an extra rinse before you eat it.

### Should I keep my laptop away from my bump?
### What about my cell phone?

Don't pull out the tin hat yet. We don't really know how or even if cellular signals or wireless connections affect your unborn child, as (drumroll, please) subjecting a fetus or pregnant woman to the risks of that research is ethically questionable.

The electromagnetic waves our devices send and receive are absorbed into our bodies in tiny amounts and, as far as we know, don't cause any harm. In high doses (like, *really* high doses), they can cause damage. Flying, the sun, and your microwave also emit electromagnetic waves, so unless you are going to live in a cave for nine months, there is no way to avoid all of it completely.

If you are worried, keep your cell phone away from your mid-section, and away from you while you sleep. Put it in airplane mode for extra points. Laptop enthusiasts, try not to use your bump as a desk, especially if your computer heats up.

# THE PREGNANCY COMMANDMENTS

## The real rules around exercise, eating, traveling, and living

I f you haven't experienced it yet, brace yourself. The moment people find out that you are pregnant, a tidal wave of differing opinions—regarding what to eat, how to deal with morning sickness, which baby items you absolutely must have, and everything else you never asked—will be unleashed.

Perhaps it's the universe preparing you for the glut of unsolicited parenting advice you'll soon receive. Perhaps there is something so tantalizing about that cute bump that people can't help but, well, want to be helpful. The point is, everyone, including your neighbors, friends, colleagues, and yes, complete strangers will have different guidance, much of it useless.

Rather than worry about every micro-decision, start by understanding the science. As we saw earlier, there's not a lot of foolproof data on how various substances or behaviors affect pregnancy, but there are certainly well-researched guidelines, and knowing them can help you decide what's best for you.

Let's start with the ins and outs of the posh aquatic habitat your baby is occupying in your abdomen.

The uterus and placenta are the two main organs involved in growing a baby. Think of the uterus as the fish tank, and the placenta as the filter and feeder. Prepregnancy, the uterus is about the size of a fist, and expands to the size of a watermelon to accommodate your growing baby. The placenta is an organ grown only during pregnancy that attaches to the wall of your uterus. It serves as the interface between mother and baby, via the umbilical cord. The placenta does many cool things, like let oxygen in and carbon dioxide out, facilitate the transfer of nutrients between you and your baby, and remove the resulting waste.

The placenta can also let in things that are not good for your baby's development. These harmful substances are known as teratogens, and they are a cause of birth defects. A teratogen's ability to cross the placenta,[1] which is dictated by molecule size, determines how harmful it is. This ability to cross is what makes the medical community so strongly against ingesting or being around known teratogens like alcohol, recreational drugs, nicotine, and carbon monoxide while you are pregnant.

So when, specifically, during the course of a pregnancy is this crossing most likely to cause issues? The short answer is, it's never a good idea to expose a growing fetus to anything that could cause harm. However, you may hear doctors say that the first trimester is when you should pay the most attention. Here's why.

Though it sounds like a time when dinosaurs roamed the earth, the teratogenic period happens in the forty-day stretch between day thirty-one and day seventy-one after your LMP. In other words, if you have a twenty-eight-day cycle, it starts three days after you've missed your period. You may or may not even know you're pregnant yet. But this period of time is when developing systems have the highest likelihood of being affected, and when many birth defects occur.[2]

The effects vary and are hard to predict. Genetics are a factor, as is the level of exposure. Some babies make it through subjection to recreational or prescribed drugs during a full pregnancy with no adverse effects, and some do not. Two to 3 percent of all pregnancies are affected by issues that occur during this period.

Now that we understand the biological mechanics, let's focus more specifically on the most important teratogens to avoid while pregnant. This includes everything from the obvious, like alcohol, to the less discussed, like prescription medications and Botox. Also below is a full list of chemicals and the products they are most commonly found in to make swapping to a clean routine easy.

One other note: Product descriptors like *organic* and *natural* across food, cosmetics, and cleaning products have absolutely no legal meaning. While it's easy to assume that these terms mean nothing artificial or synthetic is included as an ingredient, that is not always the case. If using clean products is important to you, read labels carefully or check the consumer guides on the Environmental Working Group's website.

## The vices

| Substance | Advice |
| --- | --- |
| Alcohol | Avoid during pregnancy (especially in the first trimester) |
| Caffeine | Keep total consumption under 200mg/day |
| Smoking and vaping | Avoid during conception and pregnancy |
| Cannabis | Avoid during conception and pregnancy |

## ALCOHOL

Alcohol consumption is one of the thorniest and most hotly debated subjects you'll encounter during pregnancy. It's also the most likely behavior (tied with smoking) to get you judgy looks from strangers.

What's not up for debate is that heavy drinking during pregnancy—more than two drinks per day—causes birth defects and fetal alcohol syndrome, and leads to behavioral and mental health issues later in life. Alcohol is a known teratogen, and the number of children affected by fetal alcohol syndrome spectrum disorders today is higher than the number afflicted with autism.[3]

What's less clear is the impact of more casual, moderate drinking—one to two drinks per day or less. Studies have shown that even small amounts of alcohol can cause behavioral problems, though there are so many confounding factors related to parenting styles, psychographic factors, use of other substances, and environment that it's hard to know if alcohol was in fact the root cause.

I know, I know. Your grandparents drank while pregnant and your parents are fine. Maybe your mom did and you're okay, too. European women don't give up wine. (Or do they?) Perhaps worst of all, this feels like yet another area where "better safe than sorry" is the best rationale we have, and this is more about our willingness to trust women to exercise self-control.

However, on the point of self-control, unless you want to haul a hydrometer or alcohol meter around, it's nearly impossible to know exactly how much alcohol is making it into your system, as beers and spirits have different proofs from label to label, and bartenders don't always pour consistent amounts. This issue of volume and alcohol content per serving is one reason that guidelines are and will remain conservative regardless of your willingness to self-police.

Let's get back to the science. If you rely on a literature review of medical research to reveal an indisputably "right" answer as to whether light or moderate drinking is okay, sorry to say that's not happening. If you'd like to find research that is open-ended enough to justify continuing to drink, there are studies that show light use has no known risks. However, one of the major flaws of the most frequently cited studies is that they rely on self-reported data, which means we have to rely on the subjects' memories and on their understanding of how many "drinks" they consumed. But in the words of many of the researchers who performed these studies, no evidence of harm is not the same as evidence of no harm.

As you have probably heard a thousand times, complete abstinence is what all medical professionals and organizations recommend[4] throughout pregnancy, simply because we do not understand the long-term implications. Nor are we likely to anytime soon, due to the lack of large, randomized, controlled studies, reliance on less rigorous research methods, and underlying ethical dilemmas of doing this research in the first place.

Even formerly laissez-faire European countries are now similarly conservative with their recommendations. France now advocates 100 percent abstinence during pregnancy, the UK changed its guidance from recommending that women abstain during conception and the first trimester to the entirety of pregnancy, and Italy has started warning its pregnant mothers against the possible side effects of alcohol, too.

Your taste buds change along with your sense of smell when you fall pregnant. Some women report an aversion to alcohol as an early symptom, citing a bitter taste. This can persist throughout pregnancy, so it may be that alcohol no longer tastes good anyway.

Alcohol consumption is on the decline in the US and the UK, and a growing number of tasty mocktails, shrubs, and even nonalcoholic beers are available on most menus. If you still feel self-conscious at happy hour in the early days, there are plenty of strategies to use until your news is more public. Any bartender or server will be game to help you out, so if not drinking seems tantamount to spilling the beans, get to the bar or restaurant early to place an order. Drinks like vodka soda (hold the vodka) or a sparkling beverage with a citrus or herb garnish are convincing fakes. And remember, just the act of holding something in your hand will be enough to help avert most suspicion.

Though it may seem overly conservative and unfair, in the scheme of things you sacrifice while pregnant (your body, your sleep, your ability to form coherent sentences), booze is actually a pretty small one.

*As a devout wine lover, I thought giving up alcohol would be a struggle. Surprise, surprise—I found the smell and taste of all forms of alcohol gross and vinegar-like from the early days until I gave birth, and for a while afterward, too. In the final weeks of my pregnancy, I did have a few small celebratory glasses of wine that hilariously took hours to drink. But even months after birth I found my taste for and interest in alcohol was pretty much zero.*

## CAFFEINE

Coffee and tea fans, rejoice. Repeated studies show that a small amount of caffeine is fine during pregnancy. In fact, *not* quitting cold turkey can be better. The rebound headaches caused by stopping suddenly often require medication, and those medications can be worse than just sticking with your morning cup of joe. Caffeine, along with a tall glass of water, can actually help with headaches during a time when you can't take ibuprofen or common NSAIDs.

There are downsides. Caffeine increases your blood pressure and heart rate (hey, the stimulation is the point, right?) and can cause you to feel more dehydrated. It also crosses the placenta, so your baby will feel some effect, though it doesn't cause a decrease in uterine blood flow or oxygenation.[5] And caffeine is a diuretic, so more runs to the bathroom are in your future. In very large quantities, it is linked to miscarriage, low birth weights, and infertility.

So, what is the right amount? No more than two hundred milligrams of caffeine per day is the recommendation, which is about one twelve-ounce cup of brewed coffee or two espresso shots from your favorite barista. But here come the caveats: Each brew and drink type can have differing amounts. Soft drinks and energy drinks also have caffeine in them, so if you're counting your cups, include those.

Caffeine is not just found in drinks. It's also present in chocolate and other food items that contain it or coffee flavoring, as well as in some OTC medications for pain relief, colds, and headaches.

Rather than trying to do the math every time you need a boost, figure out when your energy drops happen and when you need it the most; sip, and enjoy one drink of up to twelve ounces per day.

## SMOKING AND VAPING

This is an easy one. Smoking, whether it's cigarettes, cigars, vaping, or cigarillos, should not be done at all during pregnancy[6] or while trying to conceive. Smoking makes it harder to get pregnant and stay pregnant, it can cause premature birth or birth defects like a cleft palate, and after pregnancy, it is a risk factor for sudden infant death syndrome (SIDS).[7] Secondhand smoke is also harmful, so to reduce exposure stay out of enclosed smoky spaces and make your partner quit, too.

Though e-cigarettes don't come packed with the same myriad of harmful chemicals as traditional cigarettes, nicotine can still cause issues with your baby's lungs and brain. In other words, any nicotine delivery system is off-limits while you're pregnant.

## CANNABIS

More than 180 million people around the world use some form of cannabis, and it is increasingly available as a supplement in drinks, food, and cosmetics. Though there are eighty-five different types of cannabinoids, for purposes of this conversation we'll focus on the two most popular: tetrahydrocannabinol (THC) and cannabidiol (CBD).

THC is derived from marijuana, and is still illegal in many places around the world, though it's becoming accepted in much of the US. While it has several proven health benefits, like helping with the side effects of cancer treatment,[8] it also causes the euphoric feeling known as getting high.

CBD is primarily derived from hemp, and because it lives in a grayer legal area, it is much more widely available. CBD delivers many of the same health benefits of THC but is growing in popularity because it does so without the high. Found in everything from infused coffee and cocktails to facial creams, it's used to help with pain and stress relief. Though THC and CBD are biologically nearly identical, one atomic-level difference is responsible for their divergent effects in the body.

So why the pharmacology lesson? The Drug Enforcement Agency (DEA) requires a license to run trials involving cannabis, and limits where the strains can be sourced. Add to that the questionable ethics of testing substances on pregnant women and babies, and as with alcohol and prescription medications, you have a paucity of solid data.

Here is what we know: THC produces genetic changes in sperm and affects the pathway that helps bodily organs grow to full size as well as the genes that regulate growth during development.[9] It's not yet known whether these changes are passed down to the child. Maternal THC use has been linked to low birth weights and a higher likelihood of placement in the NICU for babies, as well as to anemia in the mothers.[10] So recreational use, and even secondhand exposure, is a bad idea while you are pregnant or trying to conceive.

The research on CBD is less clear because it has not been studied as extensively. The first CBD-powered pharmaceutical approved by the FDA, Epidiolex, gives us the best information to date on the safety of CBD for pregnant and lactating women based on two animal studies with rabbits and rats. They concluded that negative outcomes happened at 125 milligrams per kilogram, which for a 150-pound woman is 8,500 milligrams—much higher than the 10 milligrams per serving found in the commonly available tinctures and infused drinks. Doses of almost anything at that level, even prenatal vitamins, can be harmful, so it's not surprising.

More problematic if you do want to use CBD-powered products: a labeling accuracy study[11] done by the FDA reported that only twenty-six of eighty-four products labeled as CBD contained the amount claimed, and eighteen of them actually contained THC, not CBD. So even if you think a product is safe to use, due to the Wild West regulatory environment and lack of rigorous product testing, there are no guarantees.

Some practitioners are beginning to look at CBD as an alternative treatment for conditions like postpartum psychosis, as it may be more effective and safe than available prescription medications. If you find yourself presented with it as a clinical treatment option and want to confirm what you're taking is high quality, there are a few easy steps:

- Ask the company for a certificate of analysis (COA) done by an objective, third-party lab.
- Match the milligrams of CBD (and any other cannabinoids) per serving to the label's claim.
- Make sure the COA includes comprehensive testing for pesticides, molds, chemicals, and solvents—and shows they are not detected.
- The COA should be lot specific, and your product should match.

However, let it be repeated that using these products outside of medical supervision while trying to conceive, pregnant, or breastfeeding is not advisable, so always seek a professional's help.

## COSMETIC PROCEDURES

| Procedure | Advice |
|---|---|
| Injectables (fillers, Botox/ neuromodulators) | No, wait until finished with breastfeeding |
| Laser hair removal/ sclerotherapy | No, wait until finished with breastfeeding |
| Tattoos/piercings | No, wait until finished with breastfeeding |
| Facials | Yes, check ingredients and avoid salicylic and trichloroacetic acids in peels |
| Hair treatments | Yes, though consider waiting until after the first trimester and always receive treatments in well-ventilated spaces |
| Manicures/pedicures | Yes, though skip the gel polish, receive treatments in well-ventilated spaces, and ensure the salon practices safe hygiene methods and uses sterilized tools |

If you are a fan of Botox (aka neuromodulators) and fillers and facials and laser hair removal, I have good news and bad news. Well, actually, it's mostly bad news. As with cannabinoids, the ethics of testing elective cosmetic procedures on pregnant women and babies are . . . questionable, which means the number of human studies conducted is low. Frustrating, I know.

## Injectables

The main issue is whether injectable and topical compounds can cross the placental barrier to the baby. Botulinum toxin, the main ingredient in Botox, has a heavy molecular weight that makes it unlikely to do so,[12] but in FDA animal studies high doses were shown to cause low birth weight, skeletal ossification, miscarriage, premature delivery, maternal toxicity, and even death. There are no clinical studies currently that involve pregnant humans. The same goes for lactating humans, where the concern is absorption and incorporation of these products into breast milk.

If you read the labels, product manufacturers consistently state that fillers and neuromodulators are not for use by pregnant or lactating women. Allergan, the manufacturer of Botox, claims the substance should be used only "if the potential benefit justifies the potential risk to the fetus," thus putting the responsibility back on the medical provider. Even without those warnings, most medical spas and physicians will not perform elective cosmetic procedures involving any of these products on pregnant or lactating women due to the lack of conclusive data. Too much liability. If you use Botox for a medical condition, your physician will help you weigh the pros and cons of continuing its use.

## Laser hair removal and sclerotherapy

So what about laser hair removal (epilation) and sclerotherapy for those pesky pregnancy varicose veins? Both are best kept for your post-pregnancy life, as varicose veins often clear up on their own, and there is a somewhat theoretical (but real) concern around epilation because amniotic fluid may conduct galvanic current. Not to mention any hair you lasered off before pregnancy may sprout up again during those nine months.

### Tattoos and piercings

Thinking of getting inked to commemorate your new addition? Tattoos and piercings should also wait until after birth. This category also includes procedures like microblading, or any others which inject dye into the skin. The main concern is contracting an infection like hepatitis B or HIV from exposure to contaminated needles, but there is also a lack of solid research on the effects of skin dyes, especially during those critical first twelve weeks.

### Facials

Now, on to the good news! Even though you may already be sporting a rosy glow, there are plenty of ways to get safe facials. If you like chemical peels, they are primarily done with glycolic acid, lactic acid, salicylic acid, Jessner solution, and trichloroacetic acid (TCA). Of these, glycolic and lactic acid masks and peels are considered safe because their dermal penetration is negligible.

Salicylic acid, on the other hand, which is used as a topical treatment for acne, significantly penetrates the dermis and is tied to known birth defects. Jessner solution contains salicylic acid and should be avoided, and TCA should also be used with caution due to its possible dermal penetration. With the slew of facial products available these days, you should have no problem working out a solution with your aesthetician. Communicate clearly about your pregnancy, ingredients you'd like to avoid, and any concerns, and they will find a way to help you feel and look great.

### Hair treatments

More good news: Most hair treatments are considered fine, too. Research is limited when it comes to hair dyes, but the majority are non-toxic and only a small amount is absorbed into the skin. The same is true while you are breastfeeding, as dye does not enter your bloodstream.

There are many vegetable-based and low-ammonia options available. If you'd like to play it safe, substitute highlighting for full color, as the dye during highlighting is applied only to your hair, not your scalp. Many physicians suggest waiting until after the first trimester to do any treatments as an extra precaution, and to do it in a well-ventilated area with gloves if you are applying it at home. One important note on hair: Its texture, fullness, and oil content change during pregnancy (also afterward), so your normal products and treatments may not have the same effects you've grown used to.

### Manicures and pedicures

Changes in your nails are another side effect of increased hormones. Some people's nails grow more quickly and are hard as a rock; others' become brittle and split easily.

If you like to manage stress in a massage chair surrounded by celebrity gossip magazines while someone files your nails, you can continue as usual during pregnancy—with one change. To you long-lasting-polish lovers, gel is not recommended for a few reasons. Some gel polishes include methyl methacrylate monomer, which can cause allergic reactions, and the twenty-minute acetone soak to remove them has not been studied enough for the risks to be fully understood. As with any cosmetic treatment, tell your technician you are pregnant so they can exercise extra caution.

Otherwise, the rules are the same as those you'd follow while not pregnant. Any salon you visit should be well ventilated and employ safe hygiene practices, like sterilizing and cleaning tools, and have a clear health inspection record. The same goes for at-home manis and pedis: have good ventilation, clean your implements, and skip the gel.

### *Personal care products and makeup*

The beauty and cosmetics industry is notoriously unregulated in the United States, so don't expect any of your products to be labeled as not for pregnant women even if they contain the ingredients listed later in this section. There are many "natural" products that have been shown to adversely affect pregnancy and fetal development, so here's another reminder to check the labels.

Your skin is your body's biggest organ, and a few topical treatments like salicylic acid and retinoids have been shown to cause birth defects. When you review the top ingredients to avoid, where they are most commonly found, how they are labeled, and their side effects, you may question using them even after you are pregnant.

## Ingredients to avoid[13]

| Ingredient | What is it? | Labeled as |
|---|---|---|
| Retinoids | Ingredient in prescription acne and antiaging medications | Retinoic acid, retinyl palmitate, retinaldehyde, adapalene, tretinoin, tazarotene, and isotretinoin |

**Risk factors**

There's a proven link between the use of retinoids and an increased risk of birth defects for developing babies. Stop taking them several months before you plan to get pregnant.

| Ingredient | What is it? | Labeled as |
|---|---|---|
| Hydroquinone | A skin-lightening agent used to treat conditions such as chloasma and melasma | Hydroquinone, idrochinone, and quinol/1-4 dihydroxy benzene/1-4 hydroxy benzene |

**Risk factors**

As much as 45 percent of this medication is absorbed into the skin, and while no studies have yet been conducted on the effect of hydroquinone on a fetus, there is just too much of the chemical in your bloodstream after use to justify the risk.

## Ingredients to avoid (continued)

| Ingredient | What is it? | Labeled as |
|---|---|---|
| Phthalates | Chemicals added to plastics to make them more flexible and to increase the strength and effectiveness of other chemicals, such as perfume or nail polish | BzBP, DBP, DEP, DMP, or diethyl, dibutyl, or benzylbutyl phthalate |
| | **Risk factors** | |
| | Linked to everything from high blood pressure to ADHD to diabetes. New studies found connections between prenatal phthalate exposure and abnormal fetal development. Look for personal care products that are labeled "phthalate-free." | |
| Formaldehyde | A known carcinogen found in personal care products, including hair-straightening treatments, nail polish, and eyelash glue | Formaldehyde, quaternium-15, dimethyl-dimethyl (DMDM), hydantoin, imidazolidinyl urea, diazolidinyl urea, sodium hydroxymethylglycinate, and 2-bromo-2-nitropropane-1,3-diol (bromopol) |
| | **Risk factors** | |
| | Exposure is linked to spontaneous abortion, congenital malformations, and premature birth. Stick with nail polishes labeled "3-free" or "5-free," and skip the gel manis and pedis. | |

## Ingredients to avoid (continued)

| Ingredient | What is it? | Labeled as |
|---|---|---|
| Salicylic acid | Acne, exfoliating products (like combination peels), and cleansers | Salicylic acid |
| | **Risk factors** | |
| | Talk to your practitioner about topical versions, but avoid oral forms, as they can cause intracranial bleeding and other defects in the developing fetus. If you need help with sloughing or skin radiance, use products that include glycolic, lactic, or mandelic acids. | |
| Aluminum chloride hexahydrate | Common ingredient in high-powered antiperspirants | Aluminum chloride hexahydrate |
| | **Risk factors** | |
| | A common ingredient in prescription and some OTC antiperspirants, aluminum chloride hexahydrate affects the cells that produce sweat. | |
| Chemical sunscreens | Sunscreens that create a chemical reaction and work by changing UV rays into heat, then release that heat from the skin | Avobenzone, homosalate, octisalate, octocrylene, oxybenzone, octinoxate, menthyl anthranilate, and dihydroxyacetone |
| | **Risk factors** | |
| | Can cause harmful cell changes during embryonic development. Stick to mineral sunscreens and physical blockers powered by zinc oxide and titanium dioxide. | |

## Ingredients to avoid (continued)

| Ingredient | What is it? | Labeled as |
| --- | --- | --- |
| Parabens | A common preservative in cosmetics used for its antibacterial and fungicidal properties | Propyl-, butyl, isopropyl, isobutyl, and methyl-paraben |
| | **Risk factors** | |
| | Parabens are known hormone disruptors and are easily absorbed into the skin. Prenatal exposure to BPA (a paraben type) has been linked to pregnancy and childhood issues, including miscarriage, low birth weight, obesity, impaired fetal growth, and behavioral problems. | |
| Essential oils | A concentrated hydrophobic liquid containing aroma compounds from plants | Two commonly used oils are tea tree and rosemary oils |
| | **Risk factors** | |
| | Because there are so many types available, it's best to go over the safety of any individual oil with your doctor. | |

## EXERCISE

Exercise is the last thing you probably want to think about while exhausted and nauseous. And it's even harder to get motivated to get off the couch later when you feel huge. But staying active during pregnancy is important. Any exercise, even walking, can boost your mood, keeps your weight in a healthy range, and can speed up your recovery after birth. Labor and delivery are highly physical, and a strong body can make that process easier—and even shorter, in some cases. Not to mention that in the months leading up to birth, a little extra strength is helpful in carting around your growing bump.

It's not just about *your* health. Babies born to women who exercised a minimum of twenty minutes three times per week showed more localized brain activity patterns in response to sounds,[14] indicating their brains were becoming more efficient than those born to sedentary mothers. Another study demonstrated that exercising while pregnant may alter the vascular smooth tissue of infants and improve overall vascular function when they are adults.[15]

If you were active before pregnancy, keep doing what you were doing before, with a few caveats: no high-impact activities that may result in a fall or jabs to the abdomen. These include skiing and snowboarding, horseback riding, scuba diving, skating, hockey, and basketball. Your blood volume will increase by 50 percent during these nine months, which requires a lot more oxygen to maintain, so take your performance expectations down a notch. As things progress, you'll also need to make modifications to your movements, as your body just won't and can't contort itself into the same shapes anymore.

Not active before pregnancy? This isn't a call to join a gym, or the time to start training for a marathon. But unless your practitioner advises against it, try taking a few minutes (ideally a minimum of thirty) every day to walk as a start.

## GENERAL RULES OF THE ROAD

- **Abide by the talk test.** Heart rates aren't a reliable way to track whether you're going too hard, but breath is. If you can make understandable words while you exercise, you've passed the talk test.
- **Hydrate.** Water is your BFF during pregnancy, so drink a lot of it, more than you think you need.
- **Don't get overheated.** Sweating is fine, but in your first trimester especially, the surge of progesterone relaxes blood vessel walls, which lowers your blood pressure and increases your odds of light-headedness. So apologies, hot yoga enthusiasts—pregnancy is not the time for heated rooms.
- **Stretch.** Take a few minutes to warm up and cool down. Just this simple routine will help you avoid injury and maintain flexibility. Bonus points if you invest in a foam roller, which is basically like having access to an on-demand back rub. (More on foam rolling later.)
- **When it's time to stop.** If you experience any bleeding, cramping, or reduced fetal movement while exercising, it's time to stop whatever you are doing and call your doctor.

One other thing to watch: that pesky little hormone relaxin. Its job is to relax your joints, tendons, ligaments, and muscle fibers and expand your rib cage and hips in preparation for birth. Relaxin levels peak during the first trimester, and right before birth, so if you're in your favorite yoga class and able to contort even more than usual, that's why. Because relaxin promotes more flexibility, be careful and don't overstretch.

> *Exercise was the main source of sanity during my sixteen long months of on-and-off pregnancy. By stretching and staying active, I was relatively free of pain and issues, and my recovery went quickly, even after a complicated birth.*
>
> *So what did I do? The same things I did before I was pregnant. I started with strength training in the first two trimesters, modifying movements and exertion as needed. In the third, I added Pilates to help with my pelvic floor. Many times, I really didn't feel like working out and certainly couldn't maintain my previous pace. But I set a schedule, showed up, and did the best I could. And I always left feeling better than when I arrived.*

## WEIGHT GAIN

Sleeping for two, yes. Eating for two . . . sorry, no. The average baby weighs between seven and eight pounds at birth, which is sadly not large enough to justify doubling your dietary throughput. Besides, with heartburn, morning sickness, and a tiny human lounging on your digestive tract, eating large meals may not be in the cards.

The amount of weight your practitioner suggests gaining is tied to your body mass index (BMI). Invented in the 1800s by a Belgian mathematician named Adolphe Quetelet, the index is still the most common way we measure obesity. If you feel like whipping out pen and paper, BMI is your weight in kilograms over your height squared in centimeters. If you don't feel like doing metric system conversions or math, use one of the many free calculators online.

A caveat before we dive in: BMI is a terrible way to quantify a single score of one's health. The calculation does not account for muscular frames (muscle is denser than fat), so athletes are often flagged as overweight. Example: Clocking in at 240 pounds and a height of six foot two, Arnold Schwarzenegger has a BMI of 30.8, qualifying him for the obese category. Tom Cruise is five foot seven and 166 pounds, which makes his BMI 26 — overweight.

BMI also does not account for *where* a person carries weight. Even for those categorized as "normal," whether it accumulates around the hips, stomach, or butt can indicate increased risk of heart disease and diabetes. For that reason, hip and waist measurements are actually more accurate.

That helping of BMI haterade aside, it's still going to be the primary way your practitioner determines how much weight you should gain. So once you know your number, here is a guide to the recommended weight gain when carrying one baby.[16] For twins and multiples, these numbers are higher.

| Prepregnancy weight | Recommended weight gain |
|---|---|
| Underweight (BMI <18.5) | 28 to 40 lbs. |
| Normal weight (BMI 18.5 to 24.9) | 25 to 35 lbs. |
| Overweight (BMI 25 to 29.9) | 15 to 25 lbs. |
| Obese (BMI 30 or more) | 11 to 20 lbs. |

How does this translate to actual eating? If you're into counting calories, here is the additional intake per day by trimester, calculated for those in the normal weight category:

**First trimester:** no extra calories
**Second trimester:** extra 340 calories (e.g., a nice-size snack)
**Third trimester:** extra 450 calories (e.g., a sandwich)

That's right, unless you're underweight, it's not necessary to gain any weight in the first trimester. In fact, some women lose a few pounds thanks to morning sickness. So if that's you, don't stress. Weight gain during pregnancy is not linear, so don't expect to gain the same amount every week. Everyone's body is different, and if there's a reason to worry, your practitioner will let you know.

Every practitioner has a slightly different approach to these sticky dynamics. Some will share your weight each time; others will just record it without comment. If you don't want to be reminded at every appointment, ask to be told only if there's an issue. If you've had an eating disorder in the past, that's a good thing to mention at an early appointment.

So where on earth does this extra weight go? If you're retaining water, you may think it all goes to your cankles. But here is the real answer:

- **7.5 lbs.** Average full-term baby
- **7 lbs.** Stores of fat and other nutrients
- **8 lbs.** Increased blood and fluid volume
- **2 lbs.** Breasts
- **2 lbs.** Uterus
- **2 lbs.** Amniotic fluid
- **1.5 lbs.** Placenta

You will absolutely gain weight while you are pregnant. You are *supposed* to gain weight while you are pregnant. Eat healthily, and do the best you can to follow your practitioner's guidelines. Unless there is a medical reason to do so, it's not healthy to weigh yourself every day. Get help if you find yourself obsessing about every single fluctuation, and try not to compare your weight gain to friends, celebrities, or photos you find online.

*I tracked my weight once a week solely for the purpose of chiming in on this section. I did not obsess about it, and just tried to eat reasonably. My weight gain was not linear. I didn't gain any weight in the first trimester, then gained ten pounds in the second and fourteen in the third. Some weeks I gained nothing, some I lost weight, and still others I gained two or three pounds. My raging acid reflux started in the first trimester and didn't really go away until after birth, which meant I couldn't eat much at any one sitting. So I ate smaller meals and snacks throughout the day.*

*Though I wasn't counting calories and was a total carb monster, twenty-four pounds was the weight target my ob-gyn gave at my first appointment, so I was happy to end up there.*

## EATING

There are entire tomes claiming to hold the secrets to the perfect pregnancy diet. And as with everything else, "perfect" depends on whom you ask. Rather than debunking the macro, pesca-pescaterian pregnancy diet, or pushing any other specific food ideology, here's a simple truth served up hot: What works for someone else will not necessarily work for you, as everyone's bodies, preferences, and restrictions are different. All of it can and will change at least a little while you are pregnant.

Morning sickness can kill your ability to diversify beyond crackers and dry toast. Cravings may inspire strange new pairings like kimchi and chocolate cake. Acid reflux can make eating pretty much anything unpleasant. And as the weeks and months march on, meals may need to be smaller and smaller to fit in there at all.

What you eat, your baby eats, too. And eating well helps with their development and health. Knowing that makes it tempting to obsess about every single thing you put in your mouth. However, nine months is a long time and requires a more sustainable approach: paying attention and trying your best. You already know consuming pints of cookies-and-cream with reckless abandon isn't a good idea. Starting the latest fad diet, going full keto, intermittent fasting, or anything else that involves skipping meals or cutting carbs entirely is not advisable either.

A good pregnancy diet isn't that different from eating well when you are not pregnant: a mix of lean proteins, whole grains, dairy, and fruits and vegetables that come from the produce section instead of boxes and bags. If you want to stock your house with healthy choices, here are a few pregnancy power foods and their most beneficial nutrients:

## Proteins

- **Eggs**—choline, iron, and folate
- **Fish** (oily fish like salmon are best)—omega-3 fatty acids (DHA and EPA), B vitamins, potassium, and protein
- **Lean beef and pork**—iron and folate
- **Nuts**—fiber, folate, antioxidants, iron, zinc, and potassium
- **Beans and lentils**—iron, folate, zinc, and calcium

## Vegetables

- **Dark green and leafy vegetables** (kale, collard greens, spinach, asparagus, and broccoli)—antioxidants, calcium, folate, vitamin A, potassium, and fiber
- **Sweet potatoes**—packed with fiber and vitamins B6 and C, iron, potassium, and beta-carotene

## Fruits

- **Avocado**—fatty acids, fiber, potassium, copper, and vitamins C, E, and K
- **Berries**—antioxidants, fiber, and vitamin C
- **Oranges**—folate and vitamin C
- **Mangoes**—fiber and vitamins A and C
- **Pears**—folate, fiber, and potassium
- **Pomegranates**—folate, iron, protein, fiber, calcium, and vitamin K

## Whole grains

- Oatmeal—protein, fiber, and vitamin B6
- **Millet, quinoa, bulgur, and barley**—protein, fiber, antioxidants, magnesium, folate, copper, iron, and manganese
- **Brown or wild rice**—folate, potassium, calcium, manganese, and vitamin B2

## Dairy

- **Greek yogurt** (or low-sugar, high-protein alternatives)—calcium, fiber, protein, zinc, and B vitamins
- **Milk** (individually wrapped cheeses are a solid snack)—calcium, protein, iodine, potassium, and B vitamins

Hate to cook or don't know where to start? There are services that craft delightful, properly portioned meals that arrive on your doorstep ready to eat, or pre-chopped and primed to pop into the oven. If you don't mind a little cooking, make easy-to-reheat meals a few times a week so your fridge is always stocked with things you like.

Okay, fine. If there is no universally right pregnancy diet, what about the list of things you *shouldn't* eat? Hearing that deli meat and sushi are off-limits, like so many things during this experience, triggers the inevitable question *Uh, why?* The answer: They can carry harmful bacteria that cause complications and problems in your GI tract.

Here are the most common food-poisoning culprits:

- Deli meat
- Undercooked, raw, and cured meats
- Soft or unpasteurized cheeses like Brie, Camembert, and blues (unpasteurized cheeses are pretty rare

in mainstream US grocery stores, but do pop up at farmers' markets, so just check the labels)
- Pâtés and spreadable meats
- Raw eggs
- Unwashed raw produce
- High-mercury seafood (ahi tuna, shark, mackerel, tilefish, marlin)
- Unpasteurized juice or cider

Let's tackle deli meat first, since it's an odd one. Although things like roasted turkey, hot dogs, and chicken breasts are fully cooked before they're packaged or sliced, they are susceptible to a bacteria called listeria. Pregnant women's immune systems are suppressed while growing a human. While it will likely cause only a mild infection for you, listeriosis can cause serious issues for your baby, including miscarriage and stillbirth. Heating food to over 165°F kills listeria, so if you're unable to resist that turkey sandwich, pop it in the oven or microwave before eating. Sadly, listeria can be found in veggies as well, so subscribe to an electronic alert on the CDC's website if you want updates on any outbreaks.

Remember toxoplasmosis? It's not just caused by bacteria found in cat feces. You are far more likely to contract it by eating raw and undercooked meats, which include fish, shellfish, and poultry. Toxoplasmosis can cause mental disabilities and blindness for your baby, so be careful if you are a lover of rare steaks or sushi.

E. coli and salmonella are the reasons you should skip the raw cookie dough, traditional Caesar dressing, and hollandaise. E. coli causes diarrhea, resulting in dehydration, but it is rarely linked to serious issues for the baby. Salmonella is similarly more nuisance than harmful to your baby, but you should still take steps to avoid it. You can also contract salmonella through the skin of poultry and reptiles, so skip the petting zoo while pregnant, too.

So, let's recap:

- Keep your portion sizes under control (you aren't actually eating for two).
- Avoid processed foods whenever possible.
- Skip common food-poisoning culprits.
- Eat smaller, more frequent meals.
- Shoot for a mix of dairy, fat, and carbs from whole foods.
- Carry healthy snacks at all times (seriously, hunger and low blood sugar strike when you least expect it).
- **Do the best you can and don't beat yourself up over the occasional indulgence—pregnancy is a marathon, not a sprint!**

*Seriously, if you want a more specific dietary regimen, have at it with one of the thousands of plans created by celebrities, mom bloggers, and nutritionists who have all discovered what they claim to be THE ONE. However, following any of these to the letter is just not possible unless you put in a lot of work cooking, avoid going out to eat, and never find yourself in a desperate moment of pregnancy hanger.*

*Cooking is a favorite hobby of mine. But during pregnancy? Nope! The mere odor of red meat or fish sent me running to a different room. Aversions were far more plentiful than my cravings, and the unending acid reflux made it hard to eat much in one sitting, or late in the day.*

*In the first trimester, I avoided everything on the don't-eat list. But after that, if I was out for a nice meal, I occasionally indulged in a medium-rare steak or lamb and even had sushi. And though I generally ate well, there was a solid two-week phase of ice cream every night, and post–forty weeks, I devoured chocolate-chip cookies like it was my job.*

## TRAVEL LIKE A PRO

How much you enjoy getting on a plane or strapping in for a road trip while pregnant will just depend on how things are going. Generally, travel in the first trimester is tolerable but not very fun. It's ideal in the second, and increasingly uncomfortable in the third. For that reason, babymoons are best in the second trimester, when energy is at its peak and your bump is not.

Most commercial airlines in the US restrict travel after thirty-six weeks. Check with your favorite airline for their specific rules, as some actually require a doctor's note as early as twenty-eight weeks. Do the math on your departure *and* return dates. In addition to that trusty note, it's a good idea to have access to your medical records just in case you have issues while away from home.

Wondering if a pat-down is better than going through the giant scary machine? You can go through the airport security line normally throughout pregnancy. Metal detectors are fine, and though they look dangerous, so are the large body scanners. If you feel safer opting out anyway, you can step out of line and ask for a physical check.

If you do have to get on a plane, here are a few pro tips:

- **Hydrate, hydrate, hydrate.** It's easy to get dehydrated while you're pregnant even when not at thirty thousand feet, so drink plenty of water to combat the plane's low humidity.
- **Wear compression socks, get up, and stretch frequently.** For longer flights, there is a small risk of deep vein thrombosis (DVT), especially if you've had previous clotting issues or are overweight. Drawing the alphabet with your toes every hour is another way to keep things moving if you're not on the aisle and sick of climbing over your neighbor.

- **Buckle up under the bump.** Traveling during the later parts of pregnancy involves figuring out how to comfortably fasten your seat belt, which can be a challenge with your larger-than-normal midsection. Make sure you slide it under your belly and cinch.
- **Eat light.** Loading up with a big meal before you board, especially with foods that cause gas, like cruciferous vegetables and carbonated drinks, is a bad idea. Try smaller portions, and avoid salty foods.
- **Opt for more legroom.** If available, book an exit row or bulkhead seat to get a few extra inches to stretch out.

*Though I was fine to fly at twenty-seven weeks when I left, I was almost denied access to my flight home from London at twenty-nine weeks for not having a doctor's note. So please, do the math on your return date and check that particular airline's policies.*

# TO TEST, OR NOT TO TEST?

## Making sense of the menu of prenatal testing options

**Y**our baby may not be ready for the SAT, but their first tests happen before they exit the womb. And they aren't the only one under the microscope. You'll be treated to what feels like a never-ending battery of pricks, pokes, prods, and blood draws during pregnancy, too.

It's easy to jump down a rabbit hole of things that could possibly go wrong, so here's a reminder that most babies are born without any problems. Unless medically indicated, many of the testing options below are just that—options. You have full control over which tests are performed, and what information you receive. That said, unless you really hate needles (or peeing), there isn't much downside to your tests, as most are noninvasive. Most practitioners will insist you keep up with blood panels each trimester, and require gestational diabetes and group B strep (GBS) screenings at a minimum.

The bigger decision is how much information you want about your growing baby. Prenatal testing looks for abnormalities that indicate developmental or physical problems. It starts with screenings that calculate the likelihood that the baby might have a condition, and progresses as needed to diagnostic tests that provide a definitive answer. If you have no family history, are low risk, and everything looks fine, you probably won't be offered prenatal testing, though you can still opt in. If testing isn't called for and you still want to do it, insurance seldom covers it.

Some couples choose to forgo testing entirely. Others want to know every detail. Most will at least do ultrasounds, if only to get their first peeks at the baby and to learn its gender. But prenatal testing isn't perfect and can cause a lot of stress. There can be false negatives and positives, and diagnostic testing carries risks.

If you're weighing what's right for you, ask what you would do with the information you receive. Good news gives peace of mind. Bad news is more complicated. Knowing in advance that your baby will require special help or surgery at birth gives you time to plan, and in some cases the opportunity to manage conditions before the child is born. But you may be faced with decisions you never expect to make, like dealing with a result that reveals a severe or even fatal condition. If you know you would do nothing differently regardless of the results, testing may not be for you.

Don't worry—you and your partner won't navigate this process alone. Genetic counselors work with your provider to explain what's happening, and help you interpret the results should you need it.

## PRENATAL TESTING FOR BABY

### Ultrasounds

For many parents, the first ultrasound is when pregnancy starts to feel real, especially after showing friends and family your keepsake sonogram. But wait, isn't a sonogram the same thing as an ultrasound? Though the words are sometimes used interchangeably, an ultrasound is the procedure itself, and the resulting photo is the sonogram.

Inspired by such disparate phenomena as echolocation in bats and the sound waves used to detect undersea obstacles after the sinking of the *Titanic*, ultrasound first entered prenatal care in 1956. Dr. Ian Donald of Glasgow was the first to use it in obstetric practice, but it didn't catch on in the US for another twenty years.[1] It's now a standard of prenatal care around the world.

Ultrasound uses high-frequency sound waves to make images of the inside of the body. During pregnancy, the probe directs these sound waves through the cold gel on your stomach into your uterus. When the waves make contact with the fetus, they bounce back and create a picture. Ultrasound is used to make sure a baby is growing properly, to estimate gestational age, to check organ development and blood flow, and, of course, to discover the gender. Only two ultrasounds happen during a routine pregnancy—one in the first trimester and another in the second, known as the anatomy scan. If you are carrying multiples, have bleeding, or are considered high risk, more will be scheduled.

Before you get sad about the dearth of ultrasounds, remember that it is a diagnostic procedure, not a baby peep show. Skip the at-home Doppler to listen to your baby's heartbeat. It can be easy to miss fetal movement and hard to find the heartbeat. Same goes for predicting whose nose she has with 3-D and 4-D ultrasounds. The risks of too much ultrasound exposure haven't been studied, so minimizing the number you receive is best.

So what exactly are the risks of ultrasounds? At very high power, ultrasound waves can damage human tissue. We aren't sure exactly how high, because it isn't ethical to subject anyone to those levels for testing. What about radiation? X-rays and other medical imaging use ionizing radiation, which removes electrons from atoms and molecules. The nonionizing radiation used in ultrasound does not. When administered infrequently and performed in a medical context by a trained professional, ultrasounds are considered safe.[2]

Your first ultrasound usually happens between eight and ten

weeks. It confirms the fetal heartbeat, checks dating, ensures the pregnancy is happening in the uterus (as opposed to the fallopian tubes, a dangerous condition known as ectopic pregnancy), and reveals if you are (surprise!) growing more than one human. This is the only time in your pregnancy that your due date may shift slightly, as measurements of fetal age are more reliable in the first trimester than at any other time.

A second ultrasound can take place between eleven and fourteen weeks, as part of the first-trimester combined screening. Also known as the nuchal translucency screening, it combines measurements of the fluid at the base of the fetus's neck with results from a blood test to estimate the likelihood of genetic conditions like Down syndrome. The fluid in the nuchal fold is visible only during this period, while the tissue is still translucent.

The anatomy scan in the second trimester happens between eighteen and twenty weeks, and is your first real peek at your baby. During the thirty-to-forty-five-minute session, your baby's head and trunk will be measured, and the weight will be estimated. The scan also checks amniotic fluid levels and the state and location of the placenta, and the baby's kidneys, bladder, stomach, brain, spine, and sex organs. If you don't want to know the gender, tell your sonographer before they start. It's easy to see the presence (or absence) of a penis at this point.

Ultrasounds are usually only used later in pregnancy to monitor higher-risk women, so if yours is progressing without any issues, expect the anatomy scan to be your last. If you were hoping to get a preview of your baby's size and weight, measurements taken in the third trimester are not very accurate, and can be off by as many as one or two pounds. For that reason, it is not used to refine your due date late in the game.

### Cell-free DNA (cfDNA) screening

Your baby's presence isn't confined to your uterus. Just as the later explosion of toys in your house will register your child's existence, their residency in your body is evident everywhere, by way of your bloodstream. Fetal placental fragments are detectable in your blood as early as ten weeks, and are the basis for noninvasive prenatal screening (NIPS, or NIPT). It is the most recent noninvasive testing option, and is often done in combination with the first-trimester combined test.[3]

Fetal placental fragments, which match the baby's DNA, are sampled and analyzed to screen for chromosomal abnormalities. The test looks for a high number of certain DNA, as increased amounts may mean there are extra copies of those chromosomes.

### How is it done?
Blood draw

### When is it done?
Ten weeks, with results in seven to fourteen days

### What does it test?
The majority of tests screen only for three main chromosomal conditions—trisomy 13, trisomy 18, and trisomy 21 (Down syndrome)—and sex chromosome abnormalities. NIPT also reveals the baby's gender. Other genetic markers are still being evaluated for accuracy, so you probably will not see them in your results.

### Who should get it?
Anyone can get this test, and it is increasingly offered regardless of your risk factors. It is encouraged for women who have a high-risk pregnancy, are over thirty-five, or have had a previous pregnancy with a chromosomal abnormality.

### Advantages
It's a noninvasive blood test, so there is no risk of miscarriage or complication. If the results come back clean, you likely will

not need to move on to diagnostic testing. You can also elect to find out the gender months before the twenty-week anatomy scan.

### Disadvantages

Screening tests are not diagnostic, meaning they cannot tell you with 100 percent certainty if your baby is going to be affected by any of these conditions. It assigns odds based on the presence or absence of extra chromosomal matter. If the screening is positive, your doctor will suggest a CVS or amnio to confirm. There can be false positives, especially in low-risk pregnancies. If you are looking for the most data possible, CVS and amnio can diagnose hundreds of conditions; NIPT screens for only four.

## Second-trimester quadruple screening (quad screen)

The quad screen provides your baby's risk profile for certain genetic disorders and birth defects like Down syndrome and spina bifida (failure of the neural tube along the spine to close fully). If you've already cleared a first-trimester screening, it may not be offered. But in some pregnancies, findings from multiple screens are combined to improve the detection rate of some conditions.

### How is it done?

Blood draw

### When is it done?

Fifteen to twenty-two weeks

### What does it test?

Four different markers in the pregnant woman's blood: alpha-fetoprotein (AFP), estriol, inhibin A, and HCG

### Who should get it?

Women with positive first-trimester screening, or NIPT results, or anyone who started prenatal care late

### Advantages

The quad screen is noninvasive, and a negative result decreases the likelihood you will need diagnostic tests like amnio or CVS.

### Disadvantages

The quad screen does have false positives and negatives and, like all screenings, gives you the chance of a condition, not a guarantee. If you have a positive screen, you'll speak to a genetic counselor who will advise which diagnostic test is appropriate to provide a definite answer.

### *Chorionic villus sampling (CVS)*

Chorionic villi are tiny hairlike projections found in the placenta that route nutrients, oxygen, and antibodies from you to your baby. They also hold fetal cells that contain your baby's chromosomes and DNA.

The procedure removes these fetal cells from the placenta, where it attaches to the uterine wall. CVS is a conclusive diagnostic test, and can be done as early as ten weeks. It can confirm positive NIPT or NT screening results and check for inherited disorders, and serves as an earlier alternative to amniocentesis.[4]

### How is it done?

CVS can be performed two ways—transabdominally with a needle inserted through the abdomen, or transcervically, using a small tube inserted through the cervix. Using ultrasound guidance, a sample of chorionic villi are suctioned or drawn from the placenta. The procedure can be uncomfortable, and some women experience cramping for several days afterward.

### When is it done?

It's the earliest available diagnostic test, done between ten and thirteen weeks. Results can come back in a few days, or weeks, depending on how many tests are run.

### What does it test?

Hundreds of different genetic and chromosomal conditions. It also reveals the gender.

### Who should get it?

CVS is offered only if there is an increased risk of genetic or chromosomal conditions, mostly due to a positive NIPT screening or a family or medical history.

### Advantages

CVS is done earlier in pregnancy than amniocentesis and results come back quickly.

### Disadvantages

CVS carries a less than 1 percent chance of miscarriage, and transcervical CVS can cause vaginal bleeding. Rates of miscarriage between transcervical and transabdominal procedures are the same. Sometimes the sample cells are not suitable for testing, so the procedure may need to be repeated. Unlike amniocentesis, CVS cannot detect any neural tube or anatomical defects.

## *Amniocentesis*

German doctors first pioneered the technique behind amniocentesis in the 1880s to relieve excess amniotic pressure on a growing fetus.[5] The amnio hit the medical mainstream in the 1950s, and is the most well known of the prenatal diagnostic tests. It can diagnose everything from genetic abnormalities and fetal lung maturity to infection through a sample of amniotic fluid. Amniotic fluid's main job is to cushion and protect the baby in the womb, and to help regulate temperature. But it also contains fetal cells and proteins, which is the basis for the amniocentesis. It was used more frequently when there were fewer testing options, and due to the risks involved, should be used only if there are medical indications.

### How is it done?

Using ultrasound guidance, your doctor will insert a thin needle into the amniotic sac away from the baby. A small sample of amniotic fluid is withdrawn, then sent to a lab and examined for genetic abnormalities. There can be stinging and cramping during the procedure, and it can cause discomfort afterward, so you'll need to relax for the rest of the day.

### When is it done?

Typically fifteen to twenty weeks into a pregnancy with results back in two weeks.

### What does it test?

Many different birth defects and genetic conditions, from cystic fibrosis and Tay-Sachs to neural tube defects like anencephaly, which CVS cannot detect.[6]

### Who should get it?

Women with abnormal ultrasounds, genetic screenings, or lab results, previous pregnancies or children with birth defects, a high-risk pregnancy, an infection like toxoplasmosis, or a family history of genetic or birth defects. It is also done for paternity testing.

### Advantages

Amniocentesis is over 99 percent accurate in detecting genetic disorders and 90 percent accurate for neural tube defects.

## Disadvantages

Similar to CVS, there is a less than 1 percent chance of miscarriage, and rare complications like preterm labor, leaking amniotic fluid, needle injury, and infection. Sometimes the test has to be repeated if the sample cannot be accurately tested. And though it is highly accurate, amnio cannot detect every single possible condition, or the severity, so there is still a chance that even with a normal result your baby will be born with a defect the test didn't find.

## TESTS JUST FOR YOU

These tests don't come until later in your pregnancy, but in the spirit of getting the less fun stuff out of the way, and giving you an easy way to reference them later, we'll cover them all in one spot.

### Rhesus (Rh) factor blood test

Named for the rhesus monkey, which also carries the gene, Rh factor is a type of protein found on the surface of red blood cells. If you have the protein, you are Rh positive. Don't have it? You are Rh negative. Eighty-five percent of people are Rh positive, and the only way your baby can be negative is for each parent to have at least one negative factor.

An incompatibility isn't a problem for you. But it is for your baby, as your immune system will perceive the baby to be a foreign object and attack. Left unaddressed, the incompatibility can cause hemolytic anemia, which causes your baby's red blood cells to be destroyed faster than they can be replaced. It can also lead to jaundice and to liver and heart failure.[7]

This screen is usually part of the blood draw at your first prenatal visit, so the incompatibility is easy to detect and treat. If you are found to be Rh negative, you'll be given Rh immunoglobulin at twenty-eight weeks, and within seventy-two hours of birth.

### Glucose screening

File this one under gross unless you love really sweet beverages. The second-trimester glucose screening happens between twenty-four and twenty-eight weeks and checks to see if you have developed gestational diabetes. It can be done in the first trimester if you have a history of diabetes or other risk factors. The format: a blood test before and after you chug a small container of poorly flavored, very sugary water. Your blood glucose will be measured before and after the sugar bomb hits, and if the level is high, you'll move on to a three-hour glucose tolerance test. This test is similar, but requires an overnight fast. Your blood sugar is measured before you drink the same unsavory drink, and then again once an hour for three hours. If your readings are still high, you will be diagnosed with gestational diabetes.

Between 2 and 10 percent of pregnancies are affected by gestational diabetes.[8] With this diagnosis, you will be prescribed insulin or metformin, a blood sugar monitor to check your levels every few hours, a healthy diet, and regular exercise. Keeping gestational diabetes under control is important, since the condition increases your odds of having a larger-than-average baby, C-section, stillbirth, or preterm birth. And hey, learning things like the difference between good carbs and bad carbs is useful long after pregnancy is over.

Gestational diabetes typically goes away after birth, but 50 percent of those affected develop type 2 diabetes later. For that reason, your levels will be checked postdelivery, then monitored every three years.

### Group B strep (GBS)

Yes, we're *really* jumping ahead a bit with this one, but hang tight. Also, get excited, as it's the last mention of tests for a while.

Done during the third trimester, between thirty-six and thirty-eight weeks, the group B strep test is a simple swab test of the vagina and perineum. GBS is a normal bacteria in the vagina (about one in four women carry it), but it can be passed to your baby on its way out during birth.[9] If that happens, it can cause severe lung, brain, and blood infections. Left untreated, there's a one in two hundred chance of infection, and a 5 percent chance of infant death. If you are GBS positive and have a vaginal delivery, you'll be given IV antibiotics. C-section moms do not need antibiotics unless the amniotic sac has ruptured.

*Prenatal testing was my least favorite part of pregnancy. It is nearly impossible not to imagine all the things that can go wrong, even if there is no reason to suspect anything actually is. And if something goes wrong once, it's even harder.*

*Two weeks after my miscarriage, the nausea and fatigue returned with a vengeance. Inexplicably, I was pregnant again. We weren't trying, but we weren't careful either. File under "things we wish we'd known": You are especially fertile right after a miscarriage.*

*This pregnancy felt the same as the first, but with one big difference. I tried but just couldn't feel excited about it. Every trip to the bathroom was stressful—I kept looking for signs it was going to go wrong again. I also couldn't shake the feeling that something wasn't right.*

*The first hint that my sinking feeling had merit came during our first prenatal appointment. The fetal measurements were already over a week behind. The doctor cautioned that we shouldn't read too much into it, as it's tough to get accurate dating so early. I still spent most of the day afterward googling what it could mean.*

*We planned to do the NIPT at ten weeks, both because of my dreaded advanced maternal age status, and since a clear screen reduces the need for invasive diagnostic tests.*

*When the genetic counselor called to say the NIPT was positive for trisomy 18, we had no idea what it was. A quick* search revealed that it was not news we wanted. Also known as Edwards syndrome, trisomy 18 is a fatal developmental condition that often ends in stillbirth.[10]

We were devastated.

Our next step was to confirm the screening result through a CVS test. Test day was one of the worst days of our lives, especially because we were surrounded by happy pregnant bumps and new babies in the waiting room. The CVS was unpleasant (felt like being pinched from the inside), but the silent, joyless ultrasound was worse. I couldn't stop sobbing.

Our fears were confirmed a very long week later when the CVS results came back. It was indeed trisomy 18, and combined with the ultrasound findings our best-case scenario was stillbirth within just weeks or months. I talked to our genetic counselor several times just to make sure I understood every possible outcome, called a genetics expert friend to vet the efficacy of the tests, and contacted a neonatologist so that we could fully understand the condition. They all confirmed that we should take the results seriously, and that there was no possibility of a happy ending. It was over.

Terminating a wanted pregnancy, even under those circumstances, was the hardest choice I've ever had to make.

The day of the procedure, it took a full morning of waiting for my cervix to ripen; the actual dilation and curettage (D&C) procedure took only thirty minutes. The dilation was uncomfortable, but other than feeling groggy and emotionally drained, I otherwise experienced very little pain.

A few close friends stopped by that evening with dinner, hugs, and distraction. If there was a silver lining, it was that when we did eventually have a baby, he or she would come into a world full of so much love and support.

The morning after the D&C, every pregnancy symptom

*was gone. And after just a day of light spotting, it was as if the whole thing had never happened.*

*The wait time to conceive again is at least two months so hormones can disappear and the cervix can heal. As we learned before, the cycle right after a pregnancy ends can be very fertile, so this time we took precautions.*

*After our two-month hiatus, I was pregnant. Again. The first cycle we tried. Nick and I agreed not to obsess about what could go wrong and just let it be. We knew we were lucky to get pregnant so easily; now we just had to wait.*

*We cleared the NIPT screening and, since everything was normal, did not opt into any diagnostic testing. While I definitely had (many) moments of anxiety, we decided to follow the process and not seek out more information than we needed.*

*It wasn't easy getting through the first trimester. But, fortunately, this pregnancy was much easier from the start. Maybe because I had more perspective. Perhaps because I was full of so much love for the people who surrounded us while we struggled. Certainly because I had no morning sickness. Definitely because I stopped white-knuckling and trying to assert control over the process.*

*Even with many of my friends in the health community, I could find no one else who had actually been through anything similar. It was this experience more than any other that inspired me to write this book.*

## FIRST-TRIMESTER CHECKLIST

☐ Create a budget for pregnancy and the first year. Items to contemplate: maternity clothes, nursery, baby supplies, birth-related costs, childcare, and support for your recovery.

☐ Check your medicine cabinet for any beauty products that contain ingredients like salicylic acid or retinoids.

☐ Go over your supplements and medications with your practitioner (if you didn't during conception).

☐ Look into complementary practices to support your pregnancy emotionally and physically.

☐ Try to relax, eat well, hydrate, exercise as your body allows—even if it's just a quick walk.

☐ Start discussions about if, when, and how to return to work, college savings, will(s) and trust(s), and advanced healthcare directives.

☐ Talk about prenatal testing with your partner.

# The Second Trimester

You can breathe a small sigh of relief when you make it into the second trimester, first because your risk of miscarriage drops, and also because you will start feeling more like yourself (though you may not look it for long). Enjoy those deep breaths while you can, as you'll be huffing and puffing as the baby's growing size starts to crowd your lungs. In the good-news column, the spending-half-your-pregnancy-looking-and-feeling-chubby-and-bloated-but-not-actually-pregnant phase—especially if it's your first—finally comes to an end.

The second trimester is the crowd favorite, as the legion pregnancy symptoms taper off, and your bump is a cute but manageable size. It's a great time to take a babymoon and plow through tasks like putting together the nursery. You can also learn your baby's gender if you haven't already, and will feel the first flutters of movement, both of which make the whole thing feel less theoretical.

*At around twenty-two weeks I no longer looked like I'd just eaten a burrito (but all the time) and had an actual bump. Though I was still a little (okay, a lot) absentminded, my energy returned, and I could make it through a whole day (and to as late as 9 p.m., a huge accomplishment) without a nap.*

*Full disclosure: After spending two-thirds of a year stuck in the first trimester, I was not a fan of pregnancy. The exhaustion, the super smell, the night peeing—I was pretty sick of the whole thing. But then . . . the kicking started and the experience became much less abstract. There was a real, live human zooming around my abdomen like a little mango-size goldfish. A male goldfish, as it turned out. Once I stopped replaying that scene from* Alien *every time I felt a flutter, it was pretty cool.*

## SO WHAT'S HAPPENING IN THERE?

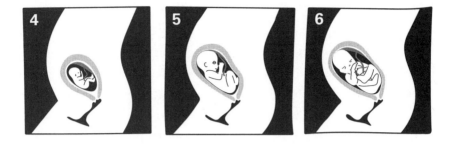

### *Month 4*

**Baby:** This month is all about moving and grooving and beginning to put on some fat. At five to six inches long, the baby is around the size of a clenched fist and is practicing breathing, sucking, and swallowing. They will start to look less like a creature from outer space and more like a human, as the ears move from the neck to the sides of the head, and their eyes get closer together. Though their body is still skinny, the baby fat you won't be able to stop pinching later begins to form along with the lungs.

**You:** Thus conclude many of the first-trimester symptoms you've grown to love. Your morning sickness should stop, the night peeing will diminish, and generally you should start to feel better. Your sex drive may also return, accompanied by new symptoms like heartburn and breathlessness. The first fetal movements, known as the quickening, are also detectable this month. They can be more like flutters or indigestion, so don't feel left out if it takes a while to discern the difference. Your swelling abdomen will finally start to look more bumplike, which means pants sans elastic will be less and less appealing by the day.

## *Month 5*

**Baby:** This is the magic month when, if you don't know already and want to, the gender will be revealed on ultrasound. Reproductive organs are forming along with a unique set of fingerprints, and your baby is just beginning to perceive the difference between light and dark—though their eyes are still fused shut. A cheese-like substance called vernix caseosa now coats their skin to protect it from pruning up in the amniotic fluid. Don't worry, it will disappear before birth. At the close of month five, your baby has nearly doubled in size, from five to six inches to eleven, and officially weighs in at about one pound.

**You:** Rejoice, you're halfway done with pregnancy! Your belly is starting to pop, and so may your belly button this month. How much you show depends entirely on your pregnancy and build—there is no standard size—so try not to compare if you're bumpin' more or less than what you see on the Internet. Pregnancy brain may cause you to forget things here and there (this symptom sticks around long after birth, sadly). The extra size and weight of the baby mean your breathlessness will increase as your lungs get pushed up, and your appetite may expand to keep up with the baby's growing demands. So may bloating and other delightful digestive issues.

## *Month 6*

**Baby:** It's time to pack on the pounds. Your baby will go from roughly one pound to two by the end of this month, and be about the size of a bowling pin. This month is all about growth—growing fat deposits, organs, bones, muscle, and even eyebrows and vocal cords. Movements will become more pronounced and easy to detect this month, and you may experience the first of many run-ins with in utero hiccups. Hearing also picks up, which means loud noises can trigger their startle reflex.

**You:** Think of month six as the sequel to month five. You'll experience many of the same changes, mostly in the form of your abdomen stretching to a basketball-like size. Your swelling size can also mean more aches and pains, and retaining fluid in your ankles and feet. Symptoms like bleeding gums, constipation, heartburn, and mysterious leg cramps can also intensify. Now is the time to watch your stress levels, as pregnancy-related hypertension can start, too.

*I had one full-on fall-on-my-face fainting spell at a crowded party as I entered the second trimester, and several other close calls in similarly warm spaces. Lesson learned that dressing in layers is the best solution to deal with the wildly vacillating pregnancy temperature swings.*

## Second-trimester symptoms and solutions

| | When does it happen? | Symptoms |
|---|---|---|
| **Skin changes** | Typically at the beginning of the second trimester, can be earlier | Linea nigra (dark line down your abdomen), melasma (dark patches on your face), stretch marks |
| **Insomnia** | Four in five women experience insomnia at some point during pregnancy. It can start during the first trimester but usually intensifies over time. | Inability to sleep through the night, waking up frequently |
| **Leg cramps and restless legs** | Can strike at any time, but more common later into pregnancy, especially common at night | Calf cramps, restless feeling in legs, inability to get comfortable |
| **Stuffy nose** | Increases throughout pregnancy, but can start anytime | Runny or bloody nose, congestion |
| **Dizziness** | Increases throughout pregnancy, but can start anytime | Light-headedness, dizziness, fainting |
| **Bleeding gums, aka pregnancy gingivitis** | Typically starts in the second trimester and persists until birth | Sensitive or bleeding gums |
| **Round ligament pain** | As your bump expands and grows, different for everyone | Crampy or achy feelings in your lower abdomen while exercising, sneezing, laughing, or getting out of bed |

| Cause | Solutions |
|-------|-----------|
| Hormonal changes cause increased melanin in the skin | They usually fade after delivery, but stay out of the sun and use sunscreen to minimize the effects. Moisturizer can help the appearance of stretch marks and related itchiness but will not prevent them. |
| Increasing bump size, night peeing, anxiety, vivid dreams, hormones, heartburn, and back pain | Invest in a body pillow, take a warm bath, or ask your partner for a massage. Pretend you're in the womb and test-drive white-noise or relaxation apps. Shorten your naps to thirty minutes or less so they don't interfere with your sleep schedule. Exercise. |
| Unclear, but thought to be related to fatigue, dehydration, or a calcium or magnesium deficiency | Exercise and walk, bath or hot shower, massage, calf raises, compression stockings, and drinking water. Ask your practitioner about taking a magnesium supplement if it's not in your prenatal vitamin. |
| Swollen mucous membranes thanks to the increased blood levels in your body | Saline rinses or drops (neti pot), humidifier, sleep with your head elevated |
| Changes in circulation | Avoid standing for long periods of time, drink plenty of fluids, and stand up slowly. |
| Hormonal changes cause increased sensitivity to the bacteria in plaque | Rinse with salt water, brush with a softer toothbrush, and keep flossing (even though it kind of sucks). |
| Muscles and ligaments stretching to support the growing uterus | Get up and down slowly, and try a belly-support band or belt. As always, listen to your body. If it happens while you exercise, or after any other specific movement, switch up the routine. |

# WHAT DO I ACTUALLY NEED TO BUY?

## Not going broke during and after pregnancy

### MATERNITY CLOTHES

Maternity attire emerged in the fourteenth century, when formerly loose and flowy dress styles that accommodated even pregnant figures evolved to be more fitted. The first known maternity dress was a style called the Adrienne, which emerged around 1600 with an empire waist and pleats designed to expand with a growing bump.[1]

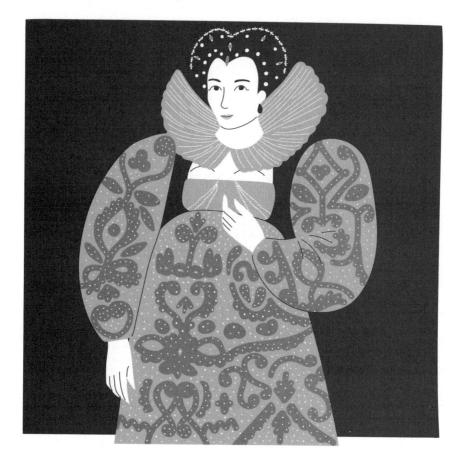

Maternity wear took a step backward in the Victorian era in the form of the maternity corset, as in those days pregnancy was considered a "condition" in need of concealment.

The notion of hiding one's "condition" persisted until 1952 when Lucille Ball famously bucked this trend. Her pregnancy was front and center in an episode of *I Love Lucy* called "Lucy Is *Enceinte*" (the word *pregnant* was deemed too vulgar for television). Lucy's on-screen style

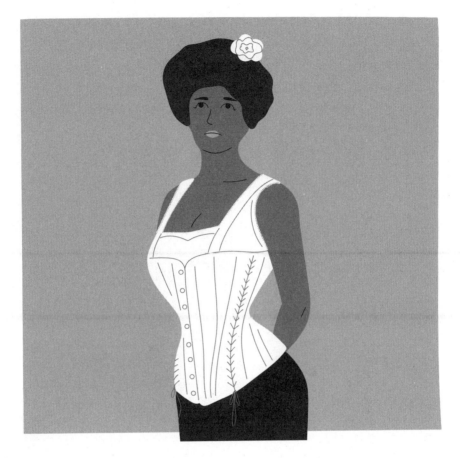

choices during her pregnancy popularized the separates trend, popular through the 1980s, in which slim skirts and pants were paired with voluminous, tentlike tops.

It wasn't until the 1990s that maternity silhouettes highlighted instead of hid changing pregnant bodies. And the ready-to-wear styles available now accommodate any size and shape your bump and body take on, and any budget or fashion need. From preggings, aka the

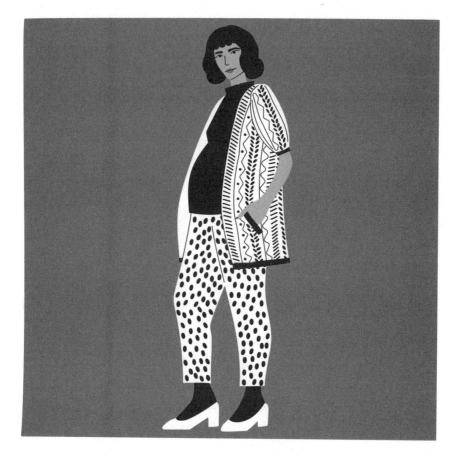

stretchy pants you'll be living in for the last months of your pregnancy, to body-con, you no longer have to live with baggy, sister-wife-style patterned dresses or fashion FOMO.

Depending how you carry, your bump might be small at the start of the second trimester, or it might already be poppin'. That bump is accompanied by bigger breasts, which means your prepregs bra size probably no longer fits. So whether you're showing or still undercover, it's time to find clothes that can comfortably handle these changes.

Most of the hard-core big-belly needs will be only for the last three to four months, so before you go down a maternity-clothes clickhole, you may be surprised at what you already have, or can get for free. Some tips:

- Peek into your closet and separate out pieces, especially dresses and shirts, that aren't super fitted, or are stretchy, longer, and have a bit of extra give. Button-down shirts are especially useful as they work open or closed, and can be thrown over dresses.
- Hit up your previously pregnant compatriots to see what they have. Someone you know may be in the middle of a purge, or at least be willing to let you borrow a few things.
- Speaking of (practically) borrowing, consignment stores, both online and offline, are full of lightly worn maternity clothes—at a major discount.

Instead of investing in an entire maternity wardrobe, which you'll want to set on fire by the time you pop, there are also services that allow you to rent clothes during your pregnancy. You can select styles and specific pieces for work, going out, lounging around, or whatever suits your life. They'll ship them out, you'll wear them as long as they fit, buy the ones you like, then send the rest back. This is especially useful for formal occasions, like that wedding when you're eight months and feel like a whale.

There are a few items worth owning. The first and most critical: pants that don't cause pain. There are a multitude of DIY ways to accommodate expanding midsections, by sewing in elastic panels or waistbands to pants you already own. But unless you are really crafty (and dedicated), at some point, you will be forced into the world of maternity pants and/or creative workarounds. And surprise! On the maternity pants front, you may never want to go back, as the proliferation of brands and options are increasingly hip and well cut, and can handle everything from the bloated, I-just-ate-a-burrito phase all the way through your first months postpartum.

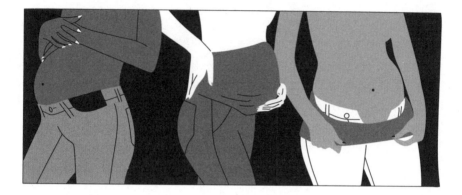

Maternity pants and key workarounds fall into a few categories: the under-bump low-rider jeans, the over-bump panel pants, and the I-can't-give-up-my-prepregnancy-pants-just-yet-elastic-band-hack.

Skirts with elastic waistbands are also useful, from loose maxi styles to more fitted cotton pencil skirts that look a bit more formal. Like many of your prepregnancy stretchy pants, you can push the waistband under or over your bump, depending on which is more comfortable.

You'll also discover the wonders of ruching, the old dressmaker's trick of gathering fabric into pleats so clothes can shrink or expand with one's body. It's a necessary (and—let's be honest—awesome) feature to allow for the growth of your bump in fitted tops and dresses.

To get you started with the basics, here is a suggested list of things you'll actually want to own. Remember that you'll continue to use many of these items postpartum and while breastfeeding (and seriously, you may never want to give up the maternity jeans):

- Maternity pants/jeans and preggings
- Several long-waisted T-shirts

- Sweaters and shirts that layer (your temperature will be all over the place)
- Nursing tanks and shirts that can pull double duty later while you're breastfeeding (get at least one black shirt that won't show breast milk leaks)
- A coat or jacket
- Pj's and loungewear that stretch
- A pair of comfortable flat shoes with some extra room (your feet can grow during pregnancy)
- Several non-underwire bras in varying sizes (it's impossible to predict your nursing-bra size, but bonus if they convert)

Okay, now clickhole away!

*My maternity wardrobe was mostly loose items I already owned, combined with consignment shop finds and a subscription box service to mix it up for the last four months. I splurged on two pairs of maternity jeans (over-the-bump style), which I loved. My all-time favorite and most complimented purchase was a pair of stretchy black pleather under-bump pants that worked equally well for professional and social occasions, and had the added bonus of making me feel like a superhero.*

## SHOPPING FOR YOUR BABY

In Finland, every mother leaves the hospital with a box of everything her new addition absolutely needs in the first thirty days of life. This tradition goes back to 1938,[2] when the box was created for low-income families to help with the terrible infant mortality rate—at that time, sixty-five out of every thousand babies died in their first year of life. To qualify, all pregnant women had to do was attend a prenatal appointment in the first trimester. The combined health and free-stuff initiative was so effective it was rolled out to the rest of the population in 1949, and continues today. In 2015, only ninety-seven babies died[3] in their first year of life across Finland's entire 5.5 million person population.

It's now possible to find Finnish-style baby boxes around the world, as they are distributed by governments in parts of Canada, Japan, Mexico, New Zealand, and Scotland. American enthusiasts have built replica versions that you can order online if you want to register for one, too.

So what's in this box anyway? Well, to start with, even the box is part of the package, as it can be the baby's first crib, provided to prevent same-bed co-sleeping. The other items include a mattress and cover, sleeping bag, undersheet, duvet, blanket, clothes in various weights and sizes, diapers and wipes, nail scissors, hairbrush, toothbrush, thermometer, diaper cream, washcloth, hooded bath towel, book and teething toy, bra pads and condoms.

### Minimum viable registry (MVR)

Though there are a few things missing, namely bottles and a pacifier (this exclusion was made to encourage breastfeeding), the reality is, for the first thirty days anyway, *babies just don't need that much stuff.* So if this configuration has been working for the mothers of Finland for the past eighty-plus years, consider their list, to borrow a software term, your minimum viable registry (MVR). We're going with the word *registry* as even if you aren't having a baby shower, it's a handy way to track what you need and what you've already purchased. A few bonus items are thrown in because, let's face it, friends and family will want to buy you some cute stuff, too.

- Infant-safe car seat
- Stroller (make sure your car seat is compatible)
- Safe place for baby to sleep (bassinet, pack 'n' play, or crib)
- Mattress, mattress cover, and a fitted sheet for crib

(skip the bumpers, pillows, and blankets—they aren't infant-safe)
- Swaddling blankets
- Diaper bag (or organizer insert)
- Pacifiers (two types)
- Changing table or pad
- Diapers (average ten changes daily, so 320 will get you through the first month)
- Wipes
- Burp cloths (you can never have too many)
- Bibs
- Clothes (newborn and 0-to-3-month sizes in case your baby comes out on the larger or longer side)
  - Onesies (wide head openings and loose legs)
  - One-piece pajamas
  - Socks
  - Hats
  - Dress-up outfits for going home, birth announcements, etc.
  - For a winter baby, two blanket sleepers, no-scratch mittens, a bunting bag, warm hat
- Rattle, teething ring, and a few other infant-safe toys
- Books
- If breastfeeding:
  - Breast pads
  - Nipple butter or lanolin
  - Breast pump
  - Pumping bra
  - Breast milk storage containers
- If formula feeding:
  - Two different bottle types
  - Newborn-friendly formula
  - Bottle-washing soap and drying rack

- Nursing pillow (if you have a C-section especially)
- Baby soap and shampoo
- Hooded baby towel/robe combo
- Grooming kit (brush, nail clippers and file, thermometer)
- First-aid kit
- Nasal aspirator
- Aquaphor (for diaper rash prevention)

### Nonessential but great to have

- Chair for feedings
- Diaper-disposal receptacle
- Floor gym/play mat (for tummy time)
- Baby monitor
- Nightlight
- White-noise machine
- Infant carrier or wrap
- Baby bathtub

### *Purchasing pro tips*

When it comes to brands and models, everyone's preferences are different. So instead of recommended individual items, what follows is the collected wisdom of parents online and interviewed to help inform your purchasing decisions.

- Newborn clothes fit only for the first few weeks (if they fit at all—hello, ten-pound babies!). Sizes are not consistent across different brands, so one company's 3 to 6 months may be another's 0 to 3. Request a variety of sizes on your registry, so your tiny human has fun clothes for the whole first year.

- Try to optimize for easy to put on clothing rather than just aesthetics. A few things to look for: kimono style or items that snap at the bottom or zip.
- Share a photo of the nursery or include (and mark "purchased") things you buy so friends who want to go off-list know what you have, and color schemes.
- To get home from the hospital, you need an infant-safe car seat. Yes, the hospital may check to make sure you have one and that it's installed correctly before allowing you to leave the premises.
- Wipe warmers are popular, but ask yourself: Do you want to haul it around when you are on the go? Getting a baby used to only warm wipes means they will be more likely to scream in public when the mobile version is cold.
- The towels and washcloths you already own are fine for your baby, too. That said, hooded towels (especially those with animal ears) are both functional and adorable!
- Get to know your baby before buying a metric ton of diapers (or anything else in bulk). Their unique needs and preferences mean some of the things you purchase just won't work.

As with maternity clothes, try to be the happy recipient of hand-me-down items, and look in consignment shops for lightly worn baby clothes. Your baby will never know the difference. Larger items like cribs, pack 'n' plays, swings, and carriers are often in play from those transitioning to the toddler years, or finally clearing out storage spaces.

One safety note on cribs: If you are inheriting a vintage model, make sure it complies with the standards the US Consumer Product Safety Commission put into place. Features like drop sides and headboard and footboard cutouts are now verboten, and the slats and corner posts should be no more than $2^3/_8$ inches apart.

*Seriously, don't buy it all in advance, and beware of different brands and their completely random sizing. We used newborn clothes for approximately one week before my son outgrew them. One European brand I love must have used mice to size their clothes, as he was too big for twelve-month onesies at just ten weeks.*

*One other thing I wish I'd known: have various pillows and portable devices to put a newborn in so you can cart them from room to room and get stuff done. My son didn't much care for being carried in a wrap or sling, so in those early weeks we depended on a fold-up minicrib and cushion that looked sort of like a pool float.*

# LET'S GET PHYSICAL

Getting to know your pelvic floor, pregnancy-friendly
exercises, and preventing aches and pains

**P**regnancy is an endurance sport. No, really—pregnant women
have the same metabolic demands as extreme athletes.[1] Unlike
ultramarathoners, you are doing the job of growing a human being
twenty-four hours a day for 280 days, with no rest days.

As we covered earlier, the best advice regarding exercising during pregnancy is: Listen to your body and avoid contact sports. And
while staying active is important, it can also be hard. Your body is
changing, your energy level (and hormones) are all over the place,
sleep isn't always great, and staying motivated while you're huge can
be a struggle.

With that in mind, this section covers the universally beneficial
movements, treatments, and knowledge that will help your body stay
physically healthy. All the exercises can be done at home with equip-
ment that costs under $20, in whatever time you can devote to it. Some
moves are doable without anyone else knowing, so Kegel, elevator,
and activate away while on conference calls, composing emails, having dinner, or sitting in traffic.

## MEET YOUR PELVIC FLOOR

Peeing when you sneeze or run might sound like something that happens only when you hit old age, just like the idea of wearing adult diapers. But all bets are off when it comes to the changes in your pelvic floor during pregnancy.

If, like most women, you're wondering, *WTF is the pelvic floor?*, they are the muscles that support the bladder, bowel, and uterus, forming a bowl shape in your pelvis. They help with everything from bathroom activities to sexual function. A strong pelvic floor is an important part of pregnancy, but also has benefits that last long after, like better sex, more bladder and bowel control, and increased spine stability.

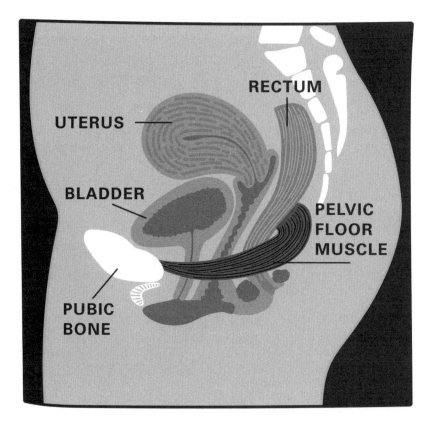

Practically speaking, a strong pelvic floor means fewer backaches, less incontinence, and a faster recovery after birth. Postpartum incontinence is pregnancy's dark little secret. Many women assume it's just part of the aftermath of vaginal birth, and that there is nothing to be done. Untrue.

A few sample exercises are included below as a gateway to this transformational work. However, working with a pelvic floor specialist starting at around thirty-four weeks through birth, and again six weeks postpartum, also provides tremendous benefit.

Referrals to a pelvic floor specialist are usually made only if you are experiencing issues like incontinence or pelvic organ prolapse. Very few midwives or ob-gyns suggest it proactively. If they do, expect to hear about it during a third-trimester appointment or at your six-week after-birth checkup. But happily, most insurance covers it, and for the low cost of a copay, you can enjoy visits before and after birth. Pelvic floor therapists are usually physical therapists, and can also help with other postpartum issues like diastasis recti (we'll get there). At a minimum, consider going in for an assessment and a one-on-one coaching session to ensure you are doing the movements correctly. This can also be done virtually if you're short on time.

### At-home pelvic floor exercises

Consider this your entrée to a stronger, healthier pelvic floor. You may recognize some of these moves from a fitness class or yoga, but they take on new meaning during pregnancy.

To perform these exercises, you'll need an elastic resistance band that fits around your thighs, and optionally a yoga mat. It's a ten-minute investment that will pay huge dividends, so try to make it a habit and do them every day.

Do two sets of ten repetitions each, with a thirty-second break between each set.

## Bird dogs

- Get in a comfortable position on your hands and knees and flatten your back.
- Engage your abs and gently lift your belly up toward your spine (think of this as drawing your baby closer to your spine with your exhale).
- Relax your baby away from your spine with each inhale.

## Bridges

- Loop the elastic band around your thighs and lie on your back with your knees bent and hip distance apart.
- Lift your hips up as high as you can, squeezing your glutes while you bridge.
- Relax, lower your hips slowly, and repeat.

## Transverse abdominis activation

- Sit on a chair with your feet flat on the floor.
- Contract your pelvic floor like you are doing a Kegel.
- Draw your belly in toward your spine.
- Hold this position for five deep breaths.
- Relax your pelvic floor and abs, repeat.

## Clamshell

- Loop the elastic band around your thighs just above the knees.
- Lie on your side on the floor or a yoga mat with your knees bent at a 90-degree angle and your hips stacked vertically on top of each other.
- Keeping your heels together, lift your top knee up to open the clamshell without moving your hips forward or backward.
- Lower your knee and repeat.

### Ride the elevator

- Do not attempt this move with a full bladder.
- While standing or sitting, imagine your pelvic floor at the ground level of a building.
- Contract your pelvic floor, then draw it up through the center of your body like an elevator going up floor by floor.
- After you've contracted fully, hold it for five seconds.
- Slowly send the elevator back down to the ground floor, one floor at a time, relax and repeat.

## STRENGTH-TRAINING MOVES

Crunches and abdominal exercises that require going from lying down straight into a seated position are off-limits while pregnant. And after the first trimester, anything that requires lying flat on your back is neither comfortable nor recommended. But you can strengthen your obliques, butt, thighs, and other core muscle groups to help with labor and recovery, all from the comfort of home.

Before you start: If you do not feel comfortable doing this without supervision, or if any of these moves hurt, stop. If you aren't currently active, talk to your doctor before jumping into a new routine.

### Cat/cow

*If you do yoga, this one will be familiar.*

- Get on your hands and knees.
- Slowly lower your head and butt and round your spine toward the ceiling.
- Return to a neutral spine position.
- Arch your back and reach the top of your head and your tailbone upward.

- Return to a neutral spine position.
- Repeat ten times.

## Squats

*You can do air squats (no weight)*
*or hold weights in each hand for this move.*

- Stand with your feet hip width apart with your toes facing forward and knees stacked above your toes.
- Bend your knees and reach back with your butt like you are sitting in a chair, keeping your chest and shoulders straight and upright.
- Stand back up.
- Repeat fifteen to twenty times.

## Side planks

*Just because you can't crunch doesn't mean*
*your abs have to be neglected for nine months.*

- Lie on your right side in a straight line.
- Make sure your elbow is directly under your shoulder, and your upper-body weight is resting on your forearm.
- Engage your obliques, gently lift your hips off the floor, and hold, maintaining a neutral spine.
- For bonus points, raise and hold your top leg while your hip is raised.
- Do two or three rounds of thirty-to-sixty-second holds on each side.

## Glute bridge

*A great one for anyone who does a lot*
*of sitting in front of a computer.*

- Lie on your back with your knees hip distance apart, knees bent.
- Engage your core, squeeze your butt, and lift your hips into a bridge.
- Hold, then return your hips to the ground one vertebra at a time.
- Repeat eight to ten times.

## Kickbacks

*There are varying degrees of difficulty*
*available with this one.*

- Get on all fours with your palms on the ground.
- Your shoulders should be directly above your palms and your knees below your hips.
- Extend one leg straight behind you, keeping your abs engaged and your spine neutral and parallel with the floor.
- Hold for three to five seconds.
- Put your leg back down to the ground and repeat by raising the other leg.
- For bonus balance points, raise the opposite arm when you raise your leg. For example, raise the right leg and left arm at the same time and hold.

## PERINEAL MASSAGE

Finally, a little relaxation after all this work! *But wait, my perineum is . . .* Yes, it's the back wall of your vagina, and part of what will later be the birth canal. The goal of perineal massage is to reduce trauma during birth by increasing flexibility and decreasing the resistance of the perineal muscles. Women who do it once or twice a week starting at week thirty-five report less pain at three months postpartum, and are less likely to require suturing after a vaginal birth.[2] A pelvic floor therapist or your doula can also walk you through a how-to, and may even offer the service during the first stages of labor.

To get started, here are the basics:

- Wash your hands and find a comfortable position (standing, sitting, or lying back) that allows you to access your perineum (after a bath or shower is a great time, as your blood vessels will be dilated, and you're already relaxed).
- Apply a small amount of unscented oil, olive oil, or lubricant (no baby oil or Vaseline!) to your thumbs, index, or middle fingers (choose one finger type).
- Insert your fingers an inch into your vagina and gently stretch and massage the back of your perineum by moving them up and down, then side to side slowly.
- Continue for up to five minutes (start slowly and work up to it), reapplying oil as needed.

*I gave pelvic floor massage my all and did it from month eight on- ward. I found the shower to be the easiest massage-parlor location, and used olive oil as a lubricant. At first, it was really awkward since reaching anything on your body (much less your perineum) is hard when you're that large, and I had no idea if I was doing it correctly. But after a few sessions things started to loosen up and I felt quite accomplished for figuring it out.*

## FOAM ROLLING

To the uninitiated, the thought of using a piece of foam to loosen up probably sounds strange. And in the third trimester, it isn't easy. There are tools like the tiger tail or self-massage stick for the final stretch if you catch the bug. But until then, foam rolling is an excellent way to give yourself a less invasive type of home massage, and release the tension in your growing body, all for as little as $5. (No, really. You can get a foam roller online for cheap.)

If you sit in front of a computer or are in your car all day or, I don't know, are carting around an extra human for nine months, your muscles develop knots and adhesions. Foam rolling provides myofascial release, which relaxes these contracted muscles. It improves the fascia, or connective tissues in the body like tendons, joints, and ligaments, and can improve blood and lymphatic circulation and even your sleep.

Foam rollers come in a variety of densities and sizes. Beginners generally like a softer, less dense roll. The truly hard-core go with versions that feature spikes. Its greatest feature is convenience. No going to a gym or spa, or waiting for your partner to offer up their services. Keep it by your bed, TV, or anywhere that provides a visual reminder and a little space.

As with any new activity, talk to your provider if your pregnancy is complicated or you are under special care. Though at first myofascial release can be uncomfortable and even a little painful, especially if you are releasing a particularly tight area, stop any movement if you are not able to balance on the roller. It's really important to be careful and gentle. YouTube has many videos that show exactly how it works if you need more in-depth guidance.

To get the most out of your rolling session, hydrate, go slow, and breathe through your movements. There are a few areas of your aching pregnant body that can really benefit from foam rolling: your outer thighs, or IT bands; your calves; and your lower back.

The basics of foam rolling:

- Sit on the floor or a yoga mat with your foam roller.
- Target a specific sore muscle and position the roller directly underneath it.
- Find a comfortable, stable position with a neutral spine.
- Use your body weight to roll over that area slowly five to ten times. If it feels good, pause and give it a moment to really sink in.

*I still keep a foam roller by my bed. I used it before and after exercise and long walks, and every night before I went to sleep. In fact, I enjoyed myofascial release so much that I went to see a massage therapist who specialized in it. She debugged a pinched nerve, unstuck my pelvis on more than one occasion, and generally helped me stay comfortable. She also won the award for care provider with the best business name: Muscle Butter.*

## AVOIDING DIASTASIS RECTI

Hold on. During pregnancy my pelvic floor is going to get trashed, you want me to use a hunk of foam to deal with back pain, and now you're telling me my abs are going to split apart?! What kind of book is this, anyway?

Sorry to be the bearer of bad news, but talk to any friends with kids, and at least a few will complain about a case of mummy tummy.

A terrifying-sounding condition called diastasis recti (DR) is the likely culprit. It happens when the connective tissue in your abdominal muscles weakens and stretches to accommodate your growing baby. This separation can result in the infamous post-pregnancy pooch, or a gap on the linea alba, the fascia that divides your six-pack.

At least 60 percent of pregnant women experience DR in varying degrees,[3] and it's not completely preventable even if you follow all of this guidance. It happens to nonpregnant people for the same reason—too much pressure on the abdominal muscles. But if you avoid certain activities and moves, your odds of getting DR go down, and if you do get it, it may not be as bad. Here are a few tips:

- **Leave the heavy lifting to someone else.** Pregnancy is not the time to become a bodybuilder. Lifting heavy weights more than twenty times per week increases the likelihood you'll develop DR.[4] If handling hefty items is a part of your job, talk to your employer. If it happens at home, unless the hefty item is your toddler, leave it to your partner.
- **Avoid crunch-like movements.** Not doing ab workouts while pregnant is intuitive. Taking your time getting out of bed will be, too, though the urge to sit straight up may not. Engaging your abs in crunch-like movements stresses your rectus abdominis.
- **Strengthen your pelvic floor and transverse abdominals.** Remember the pelvic-floor exercises earlier? The earlier you can start doing them, the better. Building a strong core will help your whole body look and feel better—during and after pregnancy.

Looking for signs? One DR telltale is abdominal doming or coning when you sit straight up from lying down, or move your shoulders off the ground like you're doing a crunch. (But seriously, stop doing crunches now!) You won't know for sure until around six weeks after birth, when your provider checks for it.

DR often goes away on its own, and if it doesn't, it is treatable (see the Fourth Trimester section for tips), so you aren't stuck with it forever. If you see a pelvic floor therapist, this is a great conversation topic, as they are usually trained to help rehabilitate DR postpartum, and will have tips to help you avoid it.

# IT'S NOT A BIRTH PLAN—IT'S PREFERENCES

## Strategizing your delivery and avoiding disappointment

**S**ome first-time mothers waltz into the labor ward with a list of demands longer than a pop star's concert rider. If you ask a nurse or doctor, there is a correlation between the length of the birth plan and likelihood of a C-section or other complications. If you ask friends with kids, most will tell you that even a textbook vaginal birth has its moments, and that there will be surprises no matter how much you plan.

Though it might seem early, the end of your second trimester is a good time to start to prepare for labor or your C-section, collect initial thoughts, and, perhaps most important, calibrate your expectations. These expectations are currently known as a birth plan.

The word *plan* is a dangerous one, as it indicates control, which, as you've hopefully figured out, during pregnancy is not really a thing. Not allowing for flexibility can lead to huge feelings of disappointment and, for some, even shame. Everything from getting a game-day epidural or needing an emergency C-section, to breastfeeding struggles or not feeling instantly bonded the first time you see your baby, can be pathways to postpartum depression.

Even if you know birth isn't something that can be managed entirely, control is still a major factor in how satisfied most women are with their birth experience.[1] This sense of control includes feeling in control of yourself in general, during contractions, and of what practitioners do to you. While pain management might affect your sense of self-control, women who feel that their practitioners listen to and care about them perceive more control over the whole experience. All of which is why it's so important to go into birth with a clear-eyed view of your options at every stage.

With that in mind, we're going to reframe your desired birth experience as birth *preferences*—not a birth *plan*. Though there are plenty of ways you can make birth feel right for you, the most critical aspect is that it ends with a healthy mom and a healthy baby. Also that the missed expectations, if and when they happen (and they will in some way), do not make you feel like you failed your transition into parenthood.

We'll start by going through the big decisions—where and how you'd like to give birth, managing pain during labor, personnel, newborn care, and contingency plans if there are any hiccups—so you feel prepared to make decisions.

A final (repeated) reminder that there is no "right" way to give birth. This process is about how you and your partner want to bring your baby into the world, allowing for any unforeseen challenges, and suiting the experience to your unique preferences. It is not about being perfect or competing for the title of most selfless human by enduring pain if you've had enough or need rest.

## REJECTING THE TERM *NATURAL BIRTH*

No doubt you've seen the term *natural childbirth* floating around. The broadest meaning is that birth is not a pathological condition, and that our bodies know what to do and need little or no outside help to do it. Adherents to the purest form of natural childbirth believe that interventions or medications of any kind add risks rather than subtract them, and some are even labeled as the "easy way out." It has also grown to mean that vaginal birth is the only "natural" method, and that C-sections are not.

Though today the natural-childbirth movement's prevailing ethos is that medical intervention is just another way of controlling women's bodies, its pioneers had very different priorities at odds with these feminist ideals.[2]

Grantly Dick-Read is heralded as the spiritual founder of the natural-childbirth movement. As an obstetrician in London in the 1920s, he explored and practiced intervention-free births; this was a revolutionary idea at a time when preventive episiotomies and mandatory sedation were increasingly common. Dick-Read penned his most well-known book, *Childbirth Without Fear*, in 1942. In it, he claimed that any pain experienced during labor was in fact psychological, and ultimately due to fear. You read that correctly. He believed that pain during labor was completely and wholly fabricated. The bulk of the book seeks to cure the underlying causes, urging practitioners to help break the fear-tension-pain cycle to make the woman relax and discipline her emotions.

Choosing to see childbirth as a zero-sum "natural" versus medicalized experience that forever determines your worth as a parent is not productive for us either as individuals or as a society that seeks to judge at every turn a process that has been repeated over 100 billion times throughout history. Adhering to the notion of "natural birth" at any cost can also be dangerous for you and your baby.

That's why we'll refer to birth as either vaginal or C-section, and medicated or unmedicated. Whether a baby comes out through your vagina or your belly, if you carried it for nine months, there is nothing unnatural about your birth, even if it's not what you planned.

## PAIN MANAGEMENT

As the American College of Obstetricians and Gynecologists points out, "there is no other circumstance in which it is considered acceptable for an individual to experience untreated severe pain, amenable to safe intervention, while under a physician's care."[3]

In other words, in the eyes of medicine, labor is sufficiently painful that in any other case, a doctor would not wait for a request or permission to offer relief.

Unless your threshold for suffering is superhuman, even with the best mental tricks and tools, at some point during labor, there will be some pain. There are nonmedical ways to manage it, like breathing, meditation, acupuncture, Lamaze, hypnobirthing, and massage. Varying levels of medication outside of an epidural are available for all the different stages of birth, too.

You may already know you'd like to go at it without any medication for as long as you can, and maybe not take any at all. Or you may want to get an epidural as soon as you arrive at the hospital. Maybe you have no clue and just want options. Trying nonmedical approaches first doesn't mean you can't also do the other—a combination of pain management methods is where most people end up.

Before we get started, here is a short public service announcement: Getting through labor without any pain relief doesn't make you a better mother, just as taking it doesn't make you a bad one. Failure for birth to go as planned, which can be as simple as requesting an epidural when you thought it was not what you wanted, can lead to postpartum depression. So instead of holding yourself to an impossible standard at an emotional, transformational time, try to put aside any judgment—external or personal. Be realistic, shut out the judgment, and choose what is right for you.

## MEDICATIONS

The Scottish doctor James Simpson first introduced anesthesia to obstetrics in 1847, first as ether and then chloroform. The real tipping point came when Dr. John Snow (famed for tracing the cause of one of London's worst cholera outbreaks to a water pump) successfully used a type of chloroform on Queen Victoria during her eighth birth[4] six years later. London's elite quickly followed her lead and the practice went mainstream.

Twilight sleep, or *Dammerschlaf*, as it was termed by its German inventors, became popular during the suffragette movement seventy years later. Its combination of morphine and scopolamine provided pain relief and had the added "bonus" of erasing the memory of birth altogether. Though American doctors were hesitant to provide this treatment (for good reason, as it resulted in psychotic behavior and nearly comatose newborns), women rose up against what they perceived as oppression and demanded it. Twilight sleep was used for decades until it finally fell out of favor in the 1950s and was replaced by an early version of today's epidural.

Labor pain medications have come a long way, and today's options range from what we all know as a standard, catheter-delivered epidural to nitrous oxide. They allow more mobility and more awareness than their previous incantations.

### The epidural

Over 60 percent of women choose to get an epidural. Women over forty are the least likely to receive one, and those under twenty are the most likely. Go figure. So what is an epidural? It's a type of anesthesia that blocks nerve impulses in the lower back, effectively decreasing feeling in the lower half of your body. The goal isn't to create a total lack of feeling, but rather minimize any painful sensations.

You can receive an epidural anytime during labor, though studies show that starting in early labor can actually prolong the process or lead to other interventions. Theoretically, you can get an epidural up until the baby actually starts crowning. The only catch: you need to be able to lie or sit still while it's placed, which can be hard during intense contractions.

There are three ways an epidural can be administered. Your hospital and physician may not offer all of them, so ask questions in your prenatal appointment if you have strong feelings.

- **Standard epidural.** A catheter is inserted into the epidural space in your spinal column and left in place so medication can be dispensed on demand.
- **Spinal block.** A single injection into the spinal fluid, the spinal block works immediately, but lasts only for one or two hours.
- **Combined spinal-epidural.** Commonly known as a walking epidural, it allows more freedom to move around during labor, though it is typically a lower dose and provides less pain relief.

With a standard epidural, an anesthesiologist numbs the area known as the epidural space, which is outside the membrane that surrounds your spinal cord and fluid. A needle is inserted and a catheter is passed through and taped on for medication delivery. Placing the catheter for an epidural can be uncomfortable but generally doesn't hurt (though the needle does look a little scary). A small amount of medicine will be dispensed as a test to check placement, and pending where you are in the labor process, a full dose will be delivered if it is deemed problem-free. The medication itself is a mix of narcotic and local anesthetic to block the pain.

Your blood pressure and the baby's heart rate will be monitored every five minutes to make sure there aren't any changes, and the effects will start ten to twenty minutes after your first dose. Afterward, you can choose to have continuous delivery through the end of labor, or control dosing through a pump that you operate as needed.

Time for upsides and downsides. The biggest upside is obvious— you will have less pain during labor if you get an epidural, though it does not take the pain to zero. As labor progresses, the amount can be dialed in to match where the pain is and how intense it becomes. Today's versions allow you to be awake and alert during labor and birth, and may allow you to get more sleep in the early stages as your cervix dilates. Because they are in less pain, many women who receive epidurals claim a more positive birth experience, as they allow more rest. And contrary to past belief, epidurals do not increase your risk of severe perineal tearing.[5]

Now, the downsides. Side effects can include backache, nausea, itching, difficulty urinating, a drop in blood pressure, and in very rare cases a severe headache. They can cause labor to last longer and can lead to more interventions like episiotomies and forceps and vacuum deliveries. You will also be hooked up to continuous monitoring for the rest of labor. The lower half of your body may be numb for a few hours after birth, which means you'll be unable to get out of bed and will need a urinary catheter. Though they are less likely to do so today, some physicians and facilities do not allow you to eat after you get an epidural, just in case you need a C-section, which means you'll be on the ice-chip diet until you deliver.

What about the effects on your newborn? Outcomes differ based on the duration of labor and other factors unique to each delivery. Babies born to mothers who chose an epidural had the same Apgar scores[6] as those who didn't. There is also no consensus related to the belief that epidurals cause difficulties with latching during early breast-feeding.[7] The majority of the medication stays in your epidural space, and little actually enters your bloodstream, so outside of a temporary dip in heart rate, the risks to your baby are minimal.

*I'll recount my full birth experience later. However, as a spoiler for that epic tale, I did not go into labor intending to get an epidural, but also did not exclude the option. I went through the safety briefing and signed the paperwork when we were admitted just in case. Without giving too much away, after ten hours of back labor, it was the most exquisite pain relief I have ever experienced. It's not without its downsides, but for me, getting an epidural allowed a few hours of sleep during a particularly long, painful, and, as you'll see, complicated labor.*

### Nitrous oxide

Used more commonly in Europe than in the US, nitrous oxide is a form of systemic pain relief that is inhaled through a face mask during labor to take the edge off. It provides immediate relief, which stops when you remove the mask. Unlike an epidural, it doesn't have any potentially detrimental effects on labor progress, and it disappears from your system quickly. However, it is not as effective in managing pain and can cause nausea, vomiting, feelings of detachment, and drowsiness.

Midwives believe one of its main benefits is that it relaxes mothers so they don't care about the pain as much, rather than the pain relief itself, since it's fairly minimal. Because you are using a mask, it also helps regulate breathing, which can help alleviate anxiety. So if you want to hold off on an epidural and still get some help, this is a safe alternative if it's offered.

*While I did end up with an epidural after exhausting all other nonmedical options during labor, I started out with just a nitrous mask, which I yelled into until I was hoarse. For me, it was less helpful for actual pain relief and more effective as a distraction.*

### Narcotics

Administered via IV or injected directly, narcotics, aka opioids, are used mostly as an alternative to the epidural. Morphine and fentanyl are two of the most common varieties, though different drugs are available pending which hospital you choose. They do not relieve as much pain as an epidural and are not usually given toward the end of labor, as they can temporarily cause neonatal respiratory depression.

Like nitrous, the side effects for you can include nausea, vomiting, breathing problems, and drowsiness. However, as all opioids cross the placenta, there are also some considerations for your baby. Though research is still not conclusive, these can range from changes in heart rate and breathing to lower early neurological scores and decreased ability to breastfeed.

## NONMEDICAL PAIN MANAGEMENT

Even if you are planning to use medications, these methods of relaxation and mindfulness can help your mind slow down and create a more pleasant experience. Techniques range from the commonly known, like meditation and aromatherapy, to those you might not know much about, like Lamaze or hypnobirthing. All of them can provide distraction and more focus during labor, and allow you to feel some amount of power over what is happening to your body.

### Acupuncture

If you tried acupuncture while trying to conceive or during pregnancy, you already know it's a branch of integrative medicine that involves pricking the skin in strategic spots with thin needles. These insertions are thought to balance energy, or qi, along pathways known as meridians in your body, helping to lessen pain and provide relaxation. Researchers don't fully understand how acupuncture works, but theories range from changing how the body perceives pain to stimulating the nervous system and production of endorphins.

Though it's believed in Chinese medicine that acupuncture can help stimulate labor, where it has proven results is during labor as a supplement to other pain relief methods. It won't shorten labor, but it has been shown to reduce the need for medication.[8] Many women also report a higher level of calm and control when asked about their birth experience later.

Though it's not standard practice, some midwives receive obstetric acupuncture training and certification. If you have one on your care team, ask if they offer it. Otherwise, some hospitals and birthing centers have acupuncturists on staff, or allow approved external acupuncturists to practice. If you enlist someone from the outside to help during labor or during your pregnancy, make sure they are well trained in obstetrical acupuncture and are not just generalists.

### Aromatherapy

Though it won't directly decrease pain, it can make the birth experience much more pleasant—for everyone. Powered by essential oils, aromatherapy has been shown to alleviate stress and improve sleep quality[9] in a range of different patients. The benefits also extend to nursing staff, who claim less stress and reduced fatigue and burnout when exposed to calming scents.[10]

Essential oils can be incorporated into a massage, misted on a pillow, or released over time with a diffuser. The top labor-recommended oils include lavender and geranium for relaxation; orange, chamomile, and mint for a lift; and clary sage to strengthen contractions.

As with all products during pregnancy, make sure the essential oils you choose are of high quality, and talk to your practitioner before you use them. And before you whip out your diffuser, make sure your hospital or birth center is okay with it in a prenatal appointment. If they are, don't forget to pack it in your labor bag!

*We went into our labor and delivery room fully loaded with lavender essential oil and a small white diffuser. While it was nice to smell during labor, and essential oils played a role later dealing with nausea, it came in most handy postpartum. Our room was the most popular on the floor less because we were good company and more because it smelled so pleasant.*

### Hypnobirthing

Hypnobirthing is a mind-body program that centers on the idea that fear of childbirth actually incites tension and physical pain. Its origins are derived from the fear-tension-pain cycle coined by the British doctor Grantly Dick-Read, the aforementioned founder of the natural-childbirth movement.

The goal of hypnobirthing is to avoid going into fight-or-flight mode during labor, by learning ways to relax. The technique utilizes positive thinking, music, affirmations, regulated breathing, and visualization to teach laboring mothers to self-hypnotize into a calm but aware state. It's thought that the increased sense of calm can help your body release contraction-friendly oxytocin and endorphins, which help blunt pain and generally make you feel good. Though hypnobirthing has not been proven to reduce pain or the number of women who request pain relief during labor,[11] it does confer a sense of control that improves postnatal anxiety and general childbirth-related fears.

If this is a route you want to pursue, involve your partner and anyone else assisting with birth. There are a number of different methods and approaches, which can be learned via an in-person class, or app, book, or video format.

### Lamaze

If you know anything about Lamaze, you likely associate it with staccato "hee hee who, hee hee who"–style huffing and puffing.

Inspired by midwife-led childbirth practices he observed in the

Soviet Union in the 1950s, the French obstetrician Dr. Fernand Lamaze created the pattern breathing–focused Lamaze technique to help laboring mothers relax during labor without medication. It's grown to encompass a more holistic view of the childbirth experience, and centers on six core tenets:

- Let labor begin on its own.
- Walk, move around, and change positions throughout labor.
- Bring a loved one, friend, or doula for continuous support.
- Avoid interventions that are not medically necessary.
- Avoid giving birth on your back and follow your body's urges to push.
- Keep mother and baby together.

The now-international Lamaze organization offers books and in-person and online classes that teach the different methods and framework for coping with pain. As with hypnobirthing, bringing your partner and birth helpers into the training process lets them know how to best support you during labor.

### Massage

No need for a professional masseuse—this is a great way to get your partner involved. Massage stimulates endorphin production through tissue manipulation, helps with relaxation, and decreases anxiety. While the current body of research is of fairly low quality, there is some proof[12] that it can provide relief and, at the very least, does no harm and is a nice way to bond with your partner.

The gate-control theory of pain is one explanation for why and how massage works during labor. Here's the idea: Non-painful sensations like gentle massage close the nerve "gates" to painful input, preventing pain from traveling to the central nervous system and brain.

Because your brain is already busy enjoying the massage, signals from contractions can't interfere and you perceive less pain as a result.

If you're working with a doula, they will share specific techniques in the months before your due date. They'll also be hands-on during birth if you like, and can step in to give your partner a break.

### Water immersion

Admit it: Labor sounds more appealing when it involves a bathtub and candles. Water immersion doesn't have to mean full-on giving birth in a tub. What it does mean is using water's magical powers to help you relax and temporarily take a load off when labor begins.

Just immersing yourself in a bathtub during the first stage of labor reduces reported pain and the need for medications.[13] The buoyancy helps take some of the stress out of your back and helps create more calming vibes. Not a bath person? Showers are also popular and come with the bonus of being able to point warm water directly at your lower back for pain relief. Some hospitals and birthing centers have a range of both available in their labor and delivery centers, so you can continue to enjoy your tub or shower time even after you leave home.

You may wonder why more people don't just go for it and give birth in a tub. The answer: Depending on whom you ask, the benefits and safety of water births vary. Water births are not for those with complicated pregnancies. They are rarely available at US hospitals, so you may not even have the option unless you want to give birth at home or in a birthing center. There's also the matter of the non-baby "discharge" in the water during birth, which means you might be sitting in poop soup.

Midwives are more pro–water birth than doctors, who are still waiting on concrete evidence before recommending the practice as an alternative to land births. (Yes, that's actually what they call it.)

But whether you're birthing by land or by sea, including hydrotherapy during early labor has no downsides and is a great complement to other relaxation techniques. It may also help reduce the amount of medication you need to manage pain.

> *My love of bathtubs is no secret. So it will come as no surprise that my only passionate birth preference was to spend as much time as I could in the water, at home in early labor and late into the process at the hospital as things progressed. Retaining the ability to bounce between the bed, yoga ball, and tub did improve the quality of my labor experience until things went a bit sideways.*

### TENS machine

More commonly used by our British friends, TENS (transcutaneous electrical nerve stimulation) is yet another weapon in the arsenal of nonmedical pain relief. It sends small pulses of electrical current through your skin into your muscles and tissue, which feels like buzzing or tingling or prickling.

How does TENS help manage labor pain? We don't really know, but assume it's a combination of distraction, endorphin release, anxiety reduction, and preventing pain signals from entering the brain.[14] The TENS device is utilized in early labor, and you can turn it up or down, toggle between different types of pulses, and change the placement based on what you need at different moments. Most of the time, it's used on the back and on acupuncture points during contractions.

The most common format is a small handheld controller connected to small pads that conduct the current to localized areas like your lower back. For those seeking active laboring options, it's highly portable—you can clip it to your gown or wear it around your neck. You'll have to give it a rest if you plan to go into the water. It is not a standard feature of hospital birthing suites, sadly. The most likely people on your care team to have a TENS machine are doulas and midwives.

*I'm not sure how effective the TENS machine was in relieving any actual pain, but I did like the way it felt. Sort of like a pleasant, very low-grade electrical shock. I found it most useful for spot treatment on the lower back and, while on full blast, as a distraction from the peak of contractions.*

## NEWBORN CARE

### Vaccines

Talking about vaccines is about as fun as discussing politics during family holidays. The need for them, the timing, the various research studies—and what kind of parent you are based on how you handle them. However, unlike many of the decisions you'll need to make related to your child's health, this one impacts everyone. Dropping immunization rates can lead to widespread outbreaks of disease, like the recent 300 percent increase in measles worldwide.

Though there has always been some resistance, the rise of the Internet amplified the multi-decade history of vaccine misinformation, most famously starting with a study by the British gastroenterologist Dr. Andrew Wakefield. In 1998, he published a paper in *The Lancet*, one of the world's most prestigious and best-known medical journals, claiming a tie between the MMR (measles, mumps, rubella) vaccine and autism. Far from a wide-ranging study involving a statistically significant, diverse set of children, it was based on a sample size of *twelve*. The findings spread like wildfire through worldwide media outlets and MMR vaccination rates plummeted. Scientists finally discredited the paper's findings in 2012, and further discovered that the data itself was falsified. Wakefield lost his license, but the damage was done.

Oprah's interview of the actress Jenny McCarthy in 2007 also contributed to the "vaccines cause autism" narrative. While promoting a book on that very subject, McCarthy claimed the MMR vaccine was responsible for her son's autism. When asked about the science that backed up her diagnosis, she said, "My science is named Evan, and he's at home. That's my science." The media blitz that followed reached fifteen to twenty million people, stoking more skepticism and bringing this idea further into the public sphere.

Even now, years after the Wakefield study was debunked, 17 percent of Americans still believe there is a tie between vaccines and autism.[15] Leading advocacy organizations like Autism Speaks are prominently pro-vaccine, pointing out that the timing of an autism diagnosis often corresponds with that of vaccinations, but isn't related. Their messaging isn't making headway either. The best pro-vaccine advocates are parents who speak in a positive way about why they value vaccines,[16] so save your shouting for Thanksgiving.

Now, on to the data. Vaccines are often cited as one of the greatest public health achievements of the twentieth century. They prevent two to three million deaths globally per year, and would prevent another 1.5 million if coverage improved. For American children born between 1994 and 2013, vaccinations will prevent 322 million illnesses, 21 million hospitalizations, and 732,000 deaths over their lifetimes, and will directly save the healthcare system $295 billion, and prevent $1.38 trillion in societal costs.[17] For all of these reasons, the WHO (World Health Organization) named vaccine hesitancy as one of the top ten threats to global health alongside HIV and ebola.[18]

The first vaccine was invented by Edward Jenner in 1796 to combat smallpox. He took material from a cowpox patient's blister and injected it into another person's skin. Not the most efficient approach, but it did pave the way for the scaled vaccine treatments to come. Diphtheria, tetanus, and pertussis were next, and in 1948 combined to become the first version of the DTP vaccine we still give today. Jonas Salk achieved rock-star status in 1955 with the polio vaccine, eliminating the fifteen thousand new cases of paralysis in the US every year. The 1960s welcomed measles, mumps, and rubella vaccinations, which combined to become MMR in 1971, just in time to celebrate the complete eradication of smallpox a year later.

Vaccines work by introducing a tiny number of antigens—the parts of a virus or bacteria that cause illness—to the body, allowing a memory immune response to develop without making a person sick. Upon the vaccine's introduction, the immune system recognizes the substance as foreign, then responds to the invading cells. It takes seven to ten days for your body to develop the desired immunologic memory, and afterward the cells remain in the body to combat future exposure.

For purposes of your birth preferences, the only vaccine decision relates to the hepatitis B shot. The rest you can wait to discuss with your pediatrician after your baby is born.

### Eye drops

Another post-birth protocol is the squirt of the antibiotic eye ointment erythromycin to prevent eye infections in newborns. If you give birth in a hospital, it is mandatory in most states. And there is no downside, as the only side effect is rare eye irritation.

Why is it important? When the baby passes through the vagina, they can be exposed to bacteria and pathogens that lead to infection, and sometimes blindness. The most common perpetrators are STDs, especially gonorrhea and chlamydia. Before you say *But there is zero chance I have an STD! Do I still have to do it?*, there are other types of bacteria like E. coli found down there, and the drops protect against that, too.

If you'd like to delay the drops until after golden-hour bonding and breastfeeding, that's fine.

### Vitamin K shot

Newborns depart the womb with low levels of vitamin K in their bodies. Vitamin K helps blood clot, so if levels are too low, it can cause dangerous bleeding in the brain or intestines. It's hard to come by in breast milk, and babies don't typically get good access to vitamin K until they start eating solid foods at around six months.

This single injection eliminates that risk; there are no side effects, and there's no compelling reason not to do it. As with the eye drops, waiting until after you've had that first bonding session to administer the shot is just fine.

### Circumcision

Circumcision's origins can be traced back to ancient religious and coming-of-age rituals in Africa, and it is still practiced in the Muslim and Jewish faiths. Roughly 33 percent of the world's male population is circumcised, and about two-thirds of those are Muslim. In the US, it rose in popularity during the Victorian era to prevent masturbation, but now only a little over half of adult males have had the procedure performed, and that number is dropping. It is even less common in Europe—20 percent across the continent and just 3.8 percent in the United Kingdom.

Circumcision is the most commonly practiced surgical procedure in human history,[19] and today's version takes just a few minutes and costs about $300.[20] In a typical circumcision, the baby receives a topical anesthetic or numbing agent; then the foreskin is clamped or separated by a plastic bell from the glans to cut off the blood supply. The surgeon then uses a scalpel to remove the foreskin and dresses the wound. Healing time is seven to ten days, and complications are minimal, just 0.4 percent in infants. That rate rises to 2 percent for older children and adults,[21] so if you're leaning yes, it is better performed on newborns.

Before we get into the pros and cons, what is the foreskin and why does it exist? On the outside, it is a natural extension of the skin of the penis. On the inside it's more like the inside of your mouth or eyelids, and secretes a natural lubricant. It contains blood vessels, neurons, skin, and a mucous membrane that covers and protects the glans, or tip of the penis. The foreskin's exact purpose and how critical it is that it be kept intact depend entirely on whom you ask. Answers range from "a worthless flap of skin whose role as protector was replaced by boxers and briefs" to "critical as a shield for the sensitive glans and full of nerve endings that increase sexual pleasure."

So why circumcise? Outside of religion, the most frequently cited reason is so that father and son match. Public health benefits are the reason most major medical organizations endorse circumcision as the standard of care. Their rationale: Epidemiological studies in sub-Saharan Africa have shown that the risk of contracting HIV drops 50 to 60 percent for circumcised heterosexual males, and 30 percent for other sexually transmitted diseases like herpes, HPV, and syphilis. We don't understand precisely why, and these numbers do not directly translate to the American population. Other health benefits include fewer urinary tract infections (UTIs), a reduction in penile cancer, and better overall cleanliness. The longtime concern that circumcised men are not able to feel as much as uncut men may not be true either. Though difficult to prove definitively, one literature review shows[22] that there is no difference in sexual pleasure or sensation attributable to circumcision status.

There are also plenty of reasons to question whether it's worth it. The number of UTIs in infants is very low, penile cancer is rare, and benefits related to STD transmission all but disappear with condom use. When it comes to pleasure, there are studies[23] that show increased sensitivity during sex in uncut men, and more pleasure for their partners with the added friction of the foreskin. Some parents opt out because they feel it's not their decision to make, that their child should decide for themselves later. Others believe it's traumatizing, though it's not clear if a newborn actually remembers the procedure. And there is further thinking that if a child was born with a foreskin, unless it's for religious reasons, there's no reason to remove it unless it's causing harm.

Like so many other decisions related to pregnancy and raising kids with no "clear-cut" (sorry!) right answer, this one is up to you and your partner to make.

### Cord blood banking

Umbilical cord fluid is loaded with stem cells, which can be used to treat immune, genetic, and neurological diseases like cancer, leukemia, and anemia.[24] Cord blood contains ten times more stem cells than bone marrow, rarely carries any infectious diseases, and is half as likely as adult stem cells to be rejected. The collection process is completely painless and takes only a few minutes. Before cutting the umbilical cord, officially separating mom and baby, the doctor clamps it, inserts a needle, and collects a minimum of 40 milliliters of blood. The cord blood is then sent to a lab or bank to be tested and stored.

Where it goes to be stored is up to you. Public cord banks make donated cord blood available to anyone, including researchers, and don't charge for storage. Private cord banks store for your family's use only, but charge fees between $1,400 and $2,300 for processing, and $95 to $125 per year to store.

So is it worth it? If you're doing it for insurance against future issues, probably not. The odds that your child will use cord blood are low, and it may be good for only fifteen years. Private banks are recommended only if there is a sibling with a medical condition that could benefit from it, or a family history of leukemia, lymphoma, sickle cell anemia, or other rare genetic disorders. However, if you'd like to contribute to research, or help build the supply, public banks are a free way to give back.

If you decide, *Yes, I want this*, cord blood banking requires advance planning. Talk to your practitioner between twenty-eight and thirty-four weeks so they can put you in touch with organizations that work with the hospital or center where you are giving birth, and ensure they have a collection process available. Four to six weeks before you're due, get in touch with a bank to coordinate the pickup.

One other consideration: If you decide to delay cord clamping, it's not always possible to bank cord blood, as the majority of the blood in the placenta and umbilical cord will go into your newborn baby's body or begin to clot. Public cord banks have minimum donation requirements, so the smaller amount may not qualify. Family banking typically imposes smaller volume limits and can be fine even if you delay. If you'd like to attempt both, just talk to your practitioner.

### Delayed cord clamping

Sorry, partner—you'll have to wait just a little longer to cut that cord. Traditionally reserved for preterm infants, delayed cord clamping is becoming more common for term newborns as well. Midwives have been advocating for delayed cord clamping for years,[25] and it's a standard of care at an increasing number of hospitals. It's easy to see why, as the benefits outweigh the known risks. But first, what is it?

The umbilical cord, the connection between the placenta and your tiny bundle, follows the baby out during delivery, right before the placenta makes its farewell. Most of the time, the cord is immediately clamped and cut within seconds of birth. With delayed cord clamping, there is no severing of that connection for several minutes, or until the cord stops pumping. Some people choose to level up further by milking, or squeezing the cord several times after it stops pulsing, to infuse the infant with all possible blood.

So what are these benefits? The majority of studies have been done only in preterm infants, but the outcomes are great.[26] These babies have higher iron levels, concentrations of hemoglobin, delivery room temperatures, blood pressure, and urine output.[27]

How about the risks? To date, there has not been enough research to prove that any past concerns like jaundice or postpartum hemorrhage are valid. But most of the studies have been done in homogenous populations, so we don't fully understand if there are nuances with more diverse ethnic backgrounds.

You will not be able to wait to cut the cord if there are any complications during birth for you or the baby. It's also sometimes not possible during a C-section birth, though you can ask.

## *Placentophagy*

Since we're talking about holistic practices, and this one is rising in popularity, let's talk about the practice of consuming your placenta after birth, or the custom's official name, placentophagy.

First, a reminder of what the placenta is and what it does. It is an organ that grows in your uterus exclusively during pregnancy to act as a filter between you and the baby. The placenta transmits oxygen and nutrients and removes waste from your baby's blood through the umbilical cord, synthesizes hormones, and is partially to blame for your increased estrogen and progesterone levels. It is expelled from your body in the first minutes after birth, as its mission of sustaining your baby during pregnancy is accomplished.

If placentophagy is a new concept for you, perhaps you are thinking, *Um, okay, why on earth would I want to eat one of my own organs?* Many mammals eat their placentas, whether to remove the scent and by-products of birth to avoid predators or for reasons we don't yet understand. While placenta has been a longtime ingredient in Chinese medicine, the first recorded instance of placentophagy was documented in 1970, in a young woman living on a commune.

Now, on to the science—or lack thereof. There are very few placentophagy studies, done with humans or animals, and there are zero done with any real scientific, double-blind, placebo-controlled rigor. The only one of the latter was a pilot study involving twenty-three women that found no significant differences in maternal iron status post–placenta consumption versus a beef placebo.[28]

There are also risks. The first is infection related to how the placenta is stored and processed.[29] Since the placenta acts as a filter, it can also contain an accumulation of potentially harmful substances, like Streptococcus agalactiae, which is a major cause of neonatal sepsis.[30] On the mental health front, ingesting placenta to prevent postpartum depression often ends up delaying women getting the medical and supportive care they need.

Long story short, the dearth of research means that we do not fully understand the known risks, that the advocacy is without physiologic basis in fact or science, and that nearly all the information out there is purely anecdotal.

If you plan to pursue placentophagy, do so with caution and visit the Association of Placenta Preparation Arts website to learn more and find a practitioner. If you are working with a doula, it may be a service they provide.

### Rooming-in versus nursery

Gone are the days of you and your first post-birth guests gazing over a field of incubators and brand-new babies behind glass. As part of new baby-friendly practices, many hospitals are now shifting from a communal nursery to rooming-in, which means your baby will hang out in your room with you after birth.

If you've had a particularly rough or long birth, the nursery is still an option even if the hospital follows baby-friendly practices. In that scenario, the baby is brought to you from the nursery for feeding, or you can walk down. But the default is to leave the baby with you to encourage breastfeeding and bonding in those early days.

Sorry, data junkies—current research does not support or refute improved rates of exclusive breastfeeding afterward,[31] as sleep is an important input into milk supply, as is the frequency of feeding in those early days. There just aren't enough high-quality trials yet.

Whether you have a vaginal birth or C-section, there are challenges to recovering from both. And while rooming-in or not doesn't have to go into your birth preferences, it can, and regardless is a good thing to understand before you arrive in your postpartum room.

## PUTTING IT ALL TOGETHER

Birth preferences capture whom you'd like to have in the room (also anyone you don't), medication preferences, what you'd like to happen after birth, and newborn care, assuming all goes smoothly. As with wit, brevity is the soul of a good list, so try to keep it to one page, and use bullets and bold anything important so it's easy for your care team to scan. Remember, these preferences can all go out the window as labor progresses, so try not to be wedded to any one thing.

The following outlines the big decisions for a hospital or birth center delivery, and includes contingency plans in case decisions need to happen on the fly. Print out a few copies so you have them on hand for different shifts (hospital providers usually rotate every twelve hours, at 7 a.m. and 7 p.m.), and in case any copies become casualties of the labor process. Take it to a prenatal appointment midway through the third trimester to discuss with your practitioner, as it's important they be able to accommodate your choices.

### Brief introduction to you and your partner, and any other birth team members

- Have fun with it, be polite, and give them a sense of your personality. After all, when you hand it over, you won't quite be yourself.
- Include phone numbers for your support team and your baby's pediatrician.
- If there is anyone you don't want present, list their names, too.

### Quick overview of obstetrical and medical history

- Number of pregnancies and births with delivery method
- List of medications, allergies, and chronic conditions

### Personal/setting the mood

- Would you like to bring music? Any lighting preferences if available?
- Do you want to labor and give birth in your own clothes?
- Whom would you like in the room during birth (partner, doula, family, etc.)?

### Medical and labor preferences for vaginal delivery

- Would you like monitoring (continuous fetal monitoring, etc.)?
- Do you want pain medication during labor and delivery? If so, which (nitrous oxide, epidural, etc.)?
- If you're unsure, would you like a saline lock placed?
- If you're at a teaching hospital, are you okay with medical students participating in your birth? (Resident participation is usually nonnegotiable.)
- Whom would you like to cut the cord?
- Would you like to delay all nonessential newborn procedures until after skin-to-skin?

### Medical preferences for cesarean delivery

- Whom would you like to be present in the OR?
- Would you like to/not like to hear the details of the procedure as they happen and have the surgical drape dropped so you can see the baby during birth?
- Do you want the cord milked?
- Do you want to hold the baby or do cheek-to-cheek immediately after birth (if possible)?

- Do you want to breastfeed within the first hour?
- Do you want your partner to do skin-to-skin if you can't?
- Do you want to delay newborn procedures until after skin-to-skin (if possible)?

## Baby

- Vitamin K shot, eye drops, hepatitis B vaccine
- Bath timing (at hospital or delay until you go home)
- Circumcision (if applicable)
- If neonatal care in the NICU is required, whom would you like to be there?

## Postpartum

- Breastfeed or formula feed?
- Rooming-in or nursery?
- Other requests related to pain management, stool-softener/laxative preferences, preserving your placenta

## SECOND-TRIMESTER CHECKLIST

☐ Finalize childcare decisions for the months after birth and your return to work.

☐ Learn about and create a draft of your birth preferences.

☐ Book a tour of your birth center.

☐ Sign up for birth class.

☐ Speak to your employer about family leave benefits (partners should do this, too).

☐ Enjoy a surge of energy and reprieve from some of your pregnancy symptoms (hopefully)!

☐ Start to put together the nursery.

# The Third Trimester

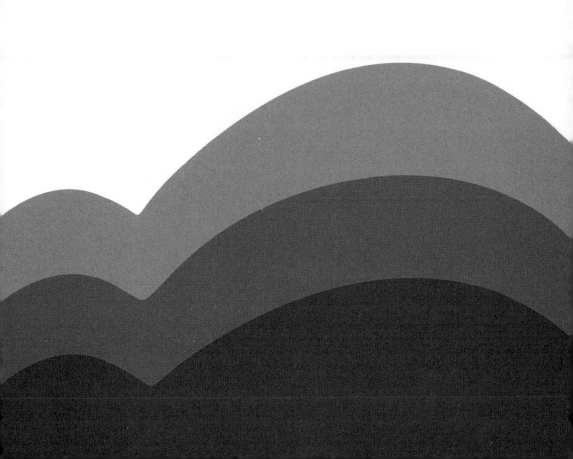

The home stretch! As the weeks wear on, your walk will become a waddle (try swinging your hips to combat this tendency), the extra weight in front means your balance will be different every day, and sleep will become increasingly difficult. You may even be able to see the outline of a foot kicking or tiny fist trying to punch its way out. While this starts off as a novelty and never stops being an amazing (if strange) feeling, when your baby is jammed up into your ribs toward the end, it can also be very uncomfortable. This discomfort also comes in the form of abdominal spasms caused by hiccups in the middle of the night, and a tiny head pressing down insistently on your bladder.

Take time to mentally and physically prepare to meet your baby, and understand what happens during birth, but don't forget you're going home after it's all over. If you need support immediately afterward, it's good to get this lined up as soon as possible.

Let's not forget about your recovery either. Baking and birthing a human is hard work, and your body will need a little extra love postpartum. Putting finishing touches on the nursery is important, but so is having a few items on hand to make you feel good.

*When I had to size up from a 32D to a 34E bra, I began to worry that my boobs were actually growing around my body and would soon connect in the back.*

*As you roll into the third trimester, you will look pregnant enough that people will no longer hesitate to say congratulations, ask how far along you are, and touch your bump. Though I was fine with friends doing it, I found this behavior by strangers mystifying. My bump was the straight-out torpedo variety, which apparently made it a very tempting target. One woman said rubbing a pregnant belly is considered good luck, which didn't really make me feel any better, or lucky. So I learned to politely let people know that they should at least ask before going for it. After all, no one ever touched my stomach when I wasn't pregnant!*

## SO WHAT'S HAPPENING IN THERE?

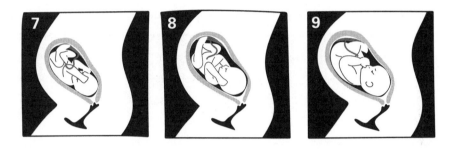

### Month 7

**Baby:** Starting in week twenty-eight, your baby will be a little over two pounds and measure around fifteen inches long. The majority of growth and development from now on will be in the brain (making connections) and packing on fat. The fat not only is helpful for temperature regulation once they join the outside world; it also means their skin will no longer be transparent. Patterns of sleeping and waking are more consistent moving forward, which means there will be an increasingly noticeable rhythm to fetal movement. By the end of the month, they will be over three pounds and sixteen inches long, getting close to their final birth length.

**You:** If you think the second trimester was crazy for growth, you ain't seen nothing yet. Strap in—your body is in for some major changes. Expect stretching, more pressure in your pelvis, and a decline back into first trimester–style fatigue as your abdomen continues to expand. Fun fact: The distance between your pubic bone and the top of your uterus in centimeters corresponds to the number of weeks you are. Your baby still has room to scoot around, which you can probably feel at times, but by the end of the month may get comfortable in a head-down position. Your dreams can intensify and feel more real, even though your sleep quality may decline. Try to focus anxious energy on what you can get done and less on everything you imagine might go wrong during birth.

### Month 8

**Baby:** Entering the ring at three to four pounds is your baby in month eight. And while they may still be a fly-weight for now, after packing on around a half pound per week, they'll end the month as a middleweight between five and six pounds and eighteen inches long. The main items on the agenda this month are practicing the basics of sucking, breathing, and—as you'll probably feel more and more frequently in your ribs with more baby and less amniotic fluid as a cushion—kicking and stretching and jabbing.

**You:** Pop! That's the sound of your belly button, which may start protruding this month. As space continues to shrink, you may become a bit more breathless as your uterus will start to crowd your lungs until the baby drops farther into your pelvis in preparation for birth. Trips to the bathroom may become increasingly long and/or complicated as digestion will continue to be sluggish, causing constipation and hemorrhoids. But one bathroom activity is here to give your poor pregnant body a break.

Spend twenty minutes in the bathtub to give yourself a little reprieve from gravity.

## Month 9

**Baby:** In the final month before their debut, your baby is packing on around half a pound per week, ending up somewhere between six and ten pounds, and measuring between nineteen and twenty-two inches. The last-minute preparations to emerge involve readying their systems for launch, building their brains, and shedding the vernix, aka that cheese-like skin coating. The cramped quarters mean that there may not be quite as much fetal movement in these final weeks, but you should still watch out for any big changes in activity.

**You:** It's almost over. Finally. You may not even notice pregnancy symptoms at this point, as you've had nine months to get used to them. Weight gain may level off, but expect vaginal discharge to pick up, your digestive tract to misbehave in all the ways you've grown accustomed to, and, once the baby's head drops, your runs to the loo to be more frequent at all times of the day and night. Braxton Hicks contractions, also known as practice contractions, may be constant in the last weeks.

## Third-trimester symptoms and solutions

| | When does it happen? | Symptoms |
|---|---|---|
| **Braxton Hicks contractions** | Can happen mid–second trimester but is most common in the third | Tightness in abdomen usually after exercise or sex |
| **Carpal tunnel syndrome** | Can happen in the second or third trimester and persist postpartum | Pain, tingling, or numbness in your hands |
| **Depression** | Though there is more focus on postpartum depression, it can start anytime during pregnancy | Loss of interest in activities you used to love, decreased ability to feel pleasure, feelings of worthlessness, fear, guilt, or suicidal thoughts |
| **Restless legs syndrome** | Can happen anytime during pregnancy, but can pick up in the third trimester, especially at night | Tingly or crawling sensation in your leg or foot while you are sitting or lying down that prevents you from feeling settled |
| **Edema** | Seventy-five percent of women experience some edema or swelling during pregnancy, though it tends to be worse toward the end of the third trimester | Swelling and fluid retention in your ankles, hands, and feet |
| **Sciatica** | Can happen in the second trimester, but is more common as your body gets bigger | Sharp or shooting pain in one or both sides of your butt or leg, numbness, difficulty walking, standing, sitting, or generally doing anything else |

| Cause | Solutions |
| --- | --- |
| Unknown but believed to help tone the uterine muscle and help blood flow to the placenta | Hydrate, and change positions. If they become painful or regular, or don't stop when you change position, call your physician as they could be a sign of preterm labor. |
| A form of edema, or built-up fluid, in your wrists that squeezes your median nerve | Treat with hand splints or ice, or use cabbage leaves as cold compresses around your wrists, acupuncture, or stretching exercises. |
| Hormonal swings, changes in your body, the major life changes happening | Speak to a loved one, schedule an appointment with your doctor, contact a mental health professional, or call a hotline. |
| Root cause is unknown, but genetic factors are suspected. Can also be triggered by iron, magnesium, or vitamin D deficiency. | Avoid caffeine late in the day. |
| Can happen in warm weather, or after too much time sitting or standing up; like stretch marks, edema is largely genetic. | Take plenty of breaks throughout the day to move, and put your feet up when you are sitting, limit your salt intake, choose comfortable shoes, and try compression socks or stockings. |
| Muscle tension and increasingly unstable joints triggered by relaxin and your expanding pelvis, the weight of the baby on your sciatic nerve. | Stretching or non-weight-bearing exercise like swimming. If you need the big guns, physical therapy, acupuncture, massage, or chiropractic care. |

## FOR PARTNERS

If you took a peek at the above third-trimester symptoms you'll know that outside of a rapidly expanding midsection, mom-to-be will be tired and moving more slowly, especially in the final weeks. Ways you can add major value: Head up final preparations to welcome the baby home, and help put together a postpartum kit for her, too.

You may be feeling anxiety around the birth, which is totally normal. That's why the chapter on birth is here—so you both have a general idea of what to expect. Make time to talk to your partner about how she would like to be supported during that experience. Your role can vary from chief labor cheerleader to running interference with family or providing a hand to squeeze.

### *Prepare for the baby*

Going shopping isn't always fun (for either of you, especially in the last weeks of pregnancy), but creating a space that is well outfitted and safe is much easier before you return home with a newborn. Though you may not care about nursery color schemes or diaper brands, whether by doing something as simple as making sure everything is assembled or taking charge of online ordering, find a way to be helpful and engaged. You'll be a hero, and the process of putting together your baby's soon-to-be space will make it all feel more real for you, too.

### *Be her advocate*

This is especially important during labor and afterward, when she is exhausted, you know, having just ejected a tiny human from her body. If you didn't help put the birth preferences together, now is an excellent time to get familiar with them. Understand exactly what she wants if everything goes well, and what to do if things go not quite as planned. If she is concerned about pain management, or really doesn't want a C-section, make sure at each turn that you are talking to the practitioners and understand the rationale for each decision.

# LIFE AFTER BIRTH

## Preparing for your baby's arrival—
## and going home after

There is no way to sugarcoat this one: The final weeks of pregnancy are tough.

Many women feel a late hit of energy and an urge to nest and clean. Others find themselves panicking about what can go wrong during birth. Still others wonder when or if their baby is ever coming out. And combined with the logistics of coordinating leave, it probably feels like the list of things you should be doing is endless.

Birth is treated a lot like a wedding. The focus is so heavily weighted toward THE BIG DAY that we often neglect to think about the full picture. Just like waking up the morning after with a marriage to maintain, you will have a tiny human whose needs are yours to fulfill for the next eighteen years after birth. Or maybe longer if they move into your basement. Not to mention, you must manage your own physical recovery. The third trimester is your time to mentally and physically prepare for birth and, more important, what comes after.

## BIRTH CLASS

Around month six, as your bump looms larger and the kicks grow more vigorous, birth becomes less abstract and more imminent. And that can be scary. But chances are, you're not the only anxious party. The idea of standing by and watching someone push a human out of their body is difficult for most people to visualize, and can end with your partner fainting if they are not mentally prepared.

Since your partner hasn't had an active physical role in pregnancy outside of moral support, foot rubs, and food fetching since their initial contribution, birth class is a great opportunity for you to bond and deal with the growing reality. And bonus: The education will give them the tools to be a great coach.

All hospitals and birth centers will have different classes on offer, ranging from marathon sessions in a single day to shorter classes that stretch out over weeks. There are even destination childbirth classes taught at resorts, if you want to add extra credit to your babymoon.

Usually classes happen in a group setting, with moms and supporters showing up together. They are taught by midwives, physicians, nurses, and doulas. In fact, if a doula is helping with your birth, sometimes they are willing to teach your class privately if your schedule is less flexible.

The goal of birth class is to provide a solid foundation to make educated choices regarding your care. The curriculum covers everything from interventions like fetal monitoring, IVs, and the circumstances in which you may need to have an unexpected C-section, to decisions regarding pain management, and even ways to add relaxation. For those who haven't seen a live birth, they will show video footage so you are mentally prepared. (Don't worry, it's less gory than you might expect.) Other classes are very hands-on, and teach breathing and massage methods.

The benefits of these classes go beyond education. They're also a way to make new parent friends. Nothing like going through the trenches together, right? This is especially useful if you're looking to pool childcare resources later, or don't have many friends with kids and are seeking potential playgroups. Welcoming a child is a big change, and being around other parents on the same timeline can provide huge emotional benefits.

Go with a smaller class size if you can, and think about how you best absorb information. If you are a hands-on learner, make sure an experiential portion is part of the package. More of an aural learner? Watching videos and listening to lectures may be the way to go.

Even if this isn't your first childbirth rodeo, the landscape and options change quickly, so signing up for a refresher isn't a bad idea. And if you're really into studying and learning, childbirth class is just the beginning. There are breastfeeding lectures, pain management classes led by anesthesiologists, infant CPR and first aid, and specialty methodologies like hypnobirthing to name a few.

## TAKE A TOUR AND PREREGISTER YOUR STAY

Whether you plan to deliver at a hospital or birthing center, labor is not the best time to get the lay of the land. Taking a pre-birth tour of the facility so you know where to go and what it's like prevents any long walks during labor, and helps you plan exactly what to bring. Partners, you can use this visit as an opportunity to scope out food availability so you know what to pack for yourself.

Outside of identifying things like the entrance and parking, here are a few questions you may want to ask on your tour:

- Will I labor and deliver in the same room?
- Are rooms private or shared?
- Is there a place for my partner to sleep in my room?
- Do you offer rooming-in so my baby can stay with me after birth versus going to a nursery?

- How long is the typical stay for a vaginal delivery versus a C-section?
- What are your visitor policies and hours?

Many facilities allow you to preregister your stay for birth, reducing the need to fill out paperwork between contractions. Others don't require it. You may be able to do this on the tour, or after one of your prenatal visits, so just ask your practitioner. You'll still need to show an insurance card and ID when you check in, but it will get you into the hands of your care team more quickly.

## PACK YOUR BAG

Plenty of people roll into the labor ward with nothing but clothes for their trip home and rely on the hospital to provide the rest, so if that's what happens, it's not a #birthfail. The only can't-give-birth-without-them items are your ID, your insurance card (if you have one), and that infant-friendly car seat. That said, consider packing a few things to help you feel human in the aftermath.

The restorative power of the first shower after birth is unreal, so at a minimum, bring the bare essentials that the hospital doesn't provide—toiletries like shampoo, soap, a toothbrush, and toothpaste, and real clothes for your departure—and call it a day. The bonus of hospital gowns is that you don't have to wash them. But getting into some of your own comfortable clothes when you're ready is really nice.

Depending on where you give birth and their specific policies, there is also room to be creative. Some moms rock out to a labor playlist using a portable speaker in a room that smells like lavender thanks to the diffuser they brought from home. Others bring their full complement of getting-ready items to help them feel more like themselves post-birth, and dress in their own cute labor-compliant gowns to avoid the open-back, butts-out hospital variety.

There is no right list, only what makes you comfortable as you welcome your new tiny human. Think of it as packing for a two- to three-day trip if you are planning to give birth vaginally, and three to four for a C-section. As a place to start, here is a mom- and labor nurse–approved list of suggestions and bonus items:

## For mom

- Insurance card and ID (must have!)
- Birth preferences printed out
- Comfortable clothing (bring washable items or things you don't mind tossing, as they may not make it through birth and early breastfeeding unscathed)
    - Loose-fitting items like yoga pants, pajamas, and nursing tops for pre- and post-birth
    - Cotton robe
    - Dark bottoms, loose top, and comfortable shoes for the ride home
    - Warm socks and/or slippers (socks need grippy bottoms—yoga or Pilates socks work well)
    - Flip-flops to wear in the shower
    - Big, comfortable postpartum underwear (you'll also have a cache of the hospital's mesh panties and giant pads)
- Eye mask and earplugs
- Travel-size toiletries (shampoo, conditioner, soap, toothbrush, toothpaste)
- Hairbrush (hair dryer if you want to feel fancy)
- Beauty products (like moisturizer, body lotion, cleansing wipes, dry shampoo, and lip balm)
- Entertainment (book, tablet, portable speaker)
- Phone charger (with a long cord, as outlets are usually far from the bed)
- Snacks

- Pillow and towels (for you and your partner—hospital varieties are thin)
- Aromatherapy diffuser and essential oils
- Toilet paper (the hospital's scratchy stuff is unsavory postpartum)
- Gifts for awesome nurses (snacks or treats are great)

### For partner

- Two wardrobe changes
- Warm hoodie or sweater
- Pajamas (or anything comfy to sleep in)
- Slippers or slip-on shoes
- Toiletries
- Entertainment (book, tablet, laptop)
- Camera and charger (with card)
- Phone charger (with extension cord)
- Sleeping bag (see what bedding the hospital or center provides while on your tour, but the standard foldout couch isn't comfortable)
- Folder to collect all the paperwork you'll accumulate

### For baby

- Infant car seat
- Mix of clothing and accessories for photos (going-home outfit is most crucial)
- Nursing pillow (if you plan to breastfeed, especially if you are planning a C-section)

*So what did I take? Answer: most of the things on this list. Friends told me about the mystical first after-birth shower, and I knew from my hospital tour that none of the accoutrements I wanted were part of the stay. So we had our previously mentioned dif-*

*fuser with lavender essential oil, a portable speaker (and multiple playlists for different moods), my favorite toiletry items, and a few inexpensive but cute hospital-like gowns for before and after. Though I shed them after a few hours of labor, it was nice to have something reasonable to put on during recovery. The item I was most relieved to have was real toilet paper, as bathroom visits are scary for a while, and hospital toilet paper is the worst.*

## CHOOSE A PEDIATRICIAN

Just like with your prenatal care, there are a range of practitioner options for your baby's medical needs. From hospital-based physicians to progressive private practices that will come to your home, you have plenty of choices to suit your priorities and needs.

Let's start with pediatricians, which are the most popular choice for infants. Just like any other medical subspecialists, they are trained to handle the specific health conditions and milestones related to tiny growing bodies. Pediatricians go through a three-year residency after their four years in medical school, then must pass a test to become officially licensed. They are recertified every seven years, and continue their education along the way so they're up to date on the latest kid-relevant literature and research.

Establishing an early relationship with a pediatrician sets the groundwork for up to twenty-one years of your child's life, as many pediatricians work from infancy all the way through adulthood. They provide preventive care, make sure growth and development are on track, and act as a primary-care physician.

It's difficult to find good online ratings and reviews for doctors, and much of what one person dislikes or loves is personal preference. You might care about their education and years in practice, philosophy on breastfeeding or sleep training, which hospital you would visit in an emergency, how they handle triaging patients to other providers when they are not available, or how they feel about prescribing antibiotics. How much time you get in each appointment is a hot-button parent issue. Each practice operates differently, and the individual slots can be as short as fifteen minutes or as long as an hour.

Many practices offer getting-to-know-you visits and interview opportunities so you can get a sense of your prospective physician's approach and personality. You may want to introduce yourself to the other partners at the practice, as over the years you will see more than one of them. If you are torn about where to start, just choose one and try a few visits when your baby joins the world to see how the physician interacts with them. You can always change later.

## REGISTER FOR A BREAST PUMP

Early human breast pumps were based on technology used in the dairy industry. The first breast pump patent was filed in 1854 by Orwell H. Needham. In his application, he describes a pump bellows connected to a nipple shield that women could press to release the flow of milk. Over the next century, other similar cow-inspired models hit the market, mostly to help infants who had difficulty nursing, or for inverted nipples. Then, in 1991, today's market leader Medela introduced the first consumer-grade electric breast pump, and the industry took off.

If you plan to breastfeed, with fairly minimal effort, you can save the $200+ you might have spent on a breast pump, as private insurers, Medicaid, and even some hospitals will provide or lend them to you at no cost. Your insurer will work with outside vendors to manage medical devices including breast pumps, so your first step is calling for that information. Next, you'll visit these vendor websites (which are named things like Yummy Mummy) to see what's available. A mix of the big pump players like Evenflo, Haakaa, Lansinoh, Medela, Philips, and Spectra should be represented.

So how do you choose? If you are a frequent traveler, or will be pumping at work, qualities like "battery-powered" and "readily available replacement parts" are critical. Noise is a concern if you plan to pump in the same room with a sleeping baby or partner, or at work.

One feature that should be mandatory in all electric pumps is the ability to toggle between stimulation and letdown modes. Stimulation does what you would assume—stimulates the flow of milk. After about two minutes, you'll manually or automatically switch into letdown or expression mode, which is designed to maximize that flow.

Looking for something more portable? There are a growing number of wearable pumps that nix the wires and bottles in favor of small, self-contained, rechargeable units that nestle into your nursing bra. They are quiet and discreet enough that you can walk around, take a call, or go out to lunch—all while pumping. Convenience and aesthetics aside, wearable versions are generally not as powerful as corded pumps, so it may take a few extra minutes to finish each session. Cost is also a consideration, since insurance does not reimburse for these models, which are typically around $400 for a double pump. However, you can use your FSA/HSA to pay for them, so it feels (slightly) less like a splurge.

The only other major thing to figure out when purchasing a breast pump is deciding which coin most closely matches the circumference of your nipple so that you order the correct-size flange. The flange is the cone-shaped pump part that seals directly onto your breast. If it doesn't fit correctly, the suction won't work, so it's important to get it right. This may take several tries, as tissue elasticity can also affect sizing. Most pumps come standard with 24mm or 27mm by default, so if you need something bigger or smaller, check with the manufacturer to make sure they make that size flange before you place your order.

If your pump arrives pre-birth, go through the sterilization and setup and play with it. There are a lot of parts to sort through and clean, and it's not the most intuitive process. Buy a few breast-pumping bras as well, so you can go fully hands-free even with a corded unit.

Most pumping bras don't require exact measurements, just a range, so you'll be fine selecting one in advance. If you'd rather skip the electronics, there are hand-expression pumps available as well.

*One of the benefits of writing this book was having an excuse to try out all the pumps. So I own one of each—corded, hand, and shove-it-in-your-bra-and-walk-around.*

*The hand pump was retired quickly, as other than building up my hand strength, it was too much work and messy. Without the portable bra version, I could see having this around as backup, though.*

*The corded version was the most powerful and fastest on full throttle. If I had to pump when I was particularly full, or in a rush, I always used it. But it was heavy, it had too many parts, and when I did use batteries, the suction was much weaker, and they drained within days.*

*The wearable pump was amazing, though not quite as unobtrusive as it purported to be. But it was much quieter than the corded version, and allowed me to do most things, including take conference calls, without thinking much about the fact that I was also pumping. The only downside: It took a while to figure out the latch, and I made a mess taking it off, then getting the bags into bottles. But it was perfect for on-the-go, as it had fewer parts to clean and was much more portable.*

## CHOOSE A NAME

Though odds are this process (or negotiation, as it is for many couples) started months ago, it's time to get serious about whittling down your options. If you did not choose to learn the gender in advance, this may involve agreeing on two different names so that no matter which way it goes, you're covered.

Some parents go into birth with a few names they like and wait to see their child before bestowing the final moniker. Others have a family name picked out before they're even pregnant. Whatever your jam, it's a permanent decision, which can feel like a lot of pressure. However, if you ask most parents later, they can't imagine any other name for their child once they give it.

You don't have to know the name at the moment of birth, though if you are in a hospital, choosing before you are discharged means it can go on the birth certificate and flow into all associated paperwork with less hassle. If you decide to go home without naming your baby, you'll have to coordinate with your State Department of Health, which is about as fun as it sounds, and adds cost. If you're giving birth at home or in a birthing center, you'll also need to get in touch with them to fill out a birth certificate.

Still riffling through books and scanning websites or need a way to trim down the options? Here are a few thoughts from the parent hive mind:

### Naming pro tips

- Look at and say the full name together to make sure it flows. Same goes for initials, and making sure they don't spell anything questionable.
- Think about possible nicknames, especially for a long or formal name. Kids' personalities don't always match.
- Same with obscenities, rhymes, and famous associations. If you don't find them, their friends at school will later.
- Have a name you love? Everyone will have an opinion, so it's up to you to decide whether to share. If you do, be prepared to stand by your choice. You are likely to be regaled with commentary from people who have an ex, family member, or frenemy with the same moniker.

- If you choose a unique spelling of a common name, know that it will be misspelled most of the time.
- Right now you are naming a baby, but your baby will spend most of their life as an adult. So be sure the name ages well.
- If you and your partner can't agree, and you plan to have more than one child, flip a coin and take turns.

## PARENTAL LEAVE

The last thing you'll want to do during your final weeks of pregnancy is obsess about every aspect of leaving work. So start planning a few months before your leave starts. Paperwork to take advantage of benefits, like FMLA and even adding your fresh family member to a health insurance plan, needs to be filled out in advance. If it's not outlined in your company benefits, call your insurance provider for specifics, but know that the typical standard is thirty to sixty days after birth to add your baby.

If your partner is planning to take leave, the below advice applies to both of you:

### Two months before birth

- Document everything so your daily duties and responsibilities at work are easy for others to access and understand.
- Start training your coworkers or replacement.
- Check in with your boss on your return-to-work timeline, and set expectations around how available you will be while out of the office.
- Stop by HR and fill out any required paperwork related to FMLA or internal policies.

- Put together a preliminary childcare plan so you don't have to scramble in the post-birth haze while you are recovering. Day care centers in large cities often have long waitlists, and you'll want to visit before you enroll your baby.
- Explore breastfeeding policies, and find out where the pumping room (if it exists) is in relation to your workspace. If there is no pumping room, ask your manager what other accommodations might be available. (A lock for your office door? A mini-fridge to store your milk?)
- Talk to other parents who have taken leave to learn their advice, any regrets, and things you may not have considered.

### Right before you leave

- Remind coworkers how often you'll be available for questions, and when you will return to the office.
- If you plan to breastfeed, block time on your calendar after your return for pumping (thirty minutes at a time, three times per day). It's easy to remove from your calendar, but harder to make time when you are getting back into things.
- Set out-of-office email and voice mail reminders.
- If you plan to shut off entirely, turn off push notifications and deactivate your email inbox on your phone so you don't get any messages.

## RETURN-TO-WORK CHILDCARE

If you don't already have a plan for long-term childcare when you return to work, you'll need a few months to figure this out. Infants are allowed in most day care centers as early as six weeks, so if you need coverage before that time, you'll need a nanny or helpful family member or friend.

### Day care

Many day care centers, especially in cities, have waiting lists for months or even years, so if this is the option you'd like, get started as early as you can.

## Pros

- Generally the most affordable option
- Set hours and calendar so less chance of schedule interruption, and gives you plenty of time to plan
- More transparency regarding their operations via online reviews and state regulations that ensure they are safe, compared with private caregivers
- More socialization at an early age

## Cons

- Most accept only full-time applicants
- Schedule has no flexibility
- More germs mean higher likelihood of kids getting sick, which means you'll need backup childcare
- Less one-on-one time from a caregiver
- Pickup and drop-off are less convenient than having someone come to your house

Family day care centers, operating in someone's home, are another option. While they can be more flexible, in-home day care is not regulated and can be hard to find.

### *Nanny or nanny share*

Having a full-time caregiver at your disposal is great for parents who need flexibility, but is also more expensive than day care. One way to offset that cost is to find another family in your area with a similarly aged child and split the expense in a nanny share.

#### Pros

- More personalized one-on-one care for your child
- Flexible schedule in case your needs change

#### Cons

- Costs are typically around three times that of day care.
- There will be more management and paperwork, as a nanny is technically your employee.

For a nanny or nanny share, it can be hard to book someone months in advance the way you would day care, so start looking three months before you need them, as they'll have a better sense of their availability. Before you commit to a candidate, do a reference check *and* in-home test to see how they are with your baby. Hearing them say they know how to give a newborn a bottle is different from seeing them do it.

### *Au pair*

Au pairs are caregivers in their late teens or early twenties who exchange childcare and other household services for room and board and a stipend. Usually they travel from a foreign country to live with a host family for one to two years.

The au pair option won't work for a newborn, as au pairs are not legally allowed to take care of infants under three months of age. But they are cheaper than nannies and have the added benefit of living in, which means a wider range of possible hours and flexibility.

### Pros

- Hugely flexible since they live in your home
- Less expensive than a nanny
- Since they typically speak another language, your child can benefit from bilingual immersion.

### Cons

- Space—you'll need a separate room in your house for them to live in.
- They will be with you for only one or two years, so it's not a long-term solution unless you are comfortable rotating through different people.

### *Staying at home*

This one may seem obvious, yet it sometimes gets forgotten. Some parents who plan to return to work do the math on childcare costs and realize they are close to (or in excess of) what they would bring home. And for some, leaving their infant in the hands of other people proves too emotionally difficult. Combined, these factors mean that even if you have every intention of going back to a full-time job, sometimes it doesn't happen.

### Pros

- You get to bond with your baby one-on-one as the primary caregiver.
- No effort spent sourcing or managing outside help.

### Cons

- If you plan to return to work later, there will be long-term impacts on your salary and career.

- It can get lonely and isolating, so it requires building a strong support network of other parents.

## POSTPARTUM PREP KIT

Hospital bag? Check. Email auto response ready to go? Check. Baby name? (Maybe) check. Frozen maxi pads and mesh panties. Huh?

If you give birth vaginally, you'll have discomfort down there for a while. C-sections have a different set of struggles but also require extra recovery care, especially the incision. If you don't want to buy now, you can snag some of these items from generous nurses before you check out of the hospital, so make friends and ask for extras.

### Must-haves

- Overnight and heavy maxi pads
- Loose-fitting underwear (stock up on hospital mesh panties, and buy your own disposables)
- Compression wrap or belly binder (helps to hold everything together while your organs return to their original locations)
- Stool softener
- Large water bottle
- Nipple ointment or lanolin (even if you're not breastfeeding, your nipples will be sore)

### Vaginal births

- Frozen-padiscle ingredients (alcohol-free witch hazel, aloe vera, spray bottle) or perineal spray
- Medicated cooling pads (Tucks or similar)
- Sitz-bath soak
- Peri, aka perineal irrigation bottle (yes, watering your perineum after birth is a thing)
- Donut pillow (especially if there was tearing)

## C-sections

- High-waisted underwear (to minimize the band rubbing against your incision)
- Breastfeeding pillow (to keep the baby's weight off your abdomen)
- Vitamin E and silicone sheeting for scar treatment

# THE BIG EVENT

## What actually happens during birth

L ike a tiny tropical storm gathering strength, your baby is finally ready to make landfall. Enough women fear pregnancy and child-birth that there is a clinical term for it—*tokophobia*.[1] Whether you watched too many medical dramas or heard horror story after horror story from friends or strangers online, it's normal to be nervous about the unknowns (and pain) of labor. Same goes for a C-section.

While it may not feel that way while it's happening, the memory of labor pain during vaginal birth is short-lived. In fact, when asked three months after labor, 90 percent of women claim to be satisfied with their experience,[2] and don't generally reference the pain at all.

What transpires during birth is influenced by whether it's your first pregnancy, the position of your baby, how you'd like to labor, medica-tion choices, and where you choose to deliver. Vaginal birth is unpre-dictable and can start anytime. Pre-scheduled C-sections are done at around thirty-eight or thirty-nine weeks.

Hopefully, building your birth preferences (and remembering that that's what they are—preferences) will help you feel confident asking questions when you need clarification or just want to understand why a course of treatment was suggested. This applies to medical staff and anyone else managing your care, as ultimately, it's your job to weigh the risks and benefits.

Rather than heighten any fears you may already have with anecdotes and birth stories (though I promise to share mine later), here is the science of birth, and how vaginal and C-section births actually work.

*Before we hit the science, one small (huge?) birth fear story.*

*At our thirty-two-week ultrasound, my son was measuring 58 percent for overall size, but his head was already over thirty-five weeks (!!!). No surprise there, as Nick's is also giant. This revelation reinforced my number one birth phobia: tearing. When it came time to discuss birth-related concerns with our doula, she reminded me that that area is meant for stretching, and then suggested I visualize his head flying out of my body while saying or thinking the phrase "My vagina is HUGE!!!" Though I am not an affirmations person, "My vagina is HUGE!!!" became my personal rallying cry every time I felt anxious.*

*One other thing: I get that the idea of not remembering or being able to describe labor pain sounds unbelievable. I didn't believe it before birth either. But even a week afterward I had flashes but could not actually articulate it other than to say labor hurt. A lot. Perhaps the memory lapse is nature's way of ensuring we do it more than once?*

## VAGINAL BIRTH

Your baby's arrival has been marked on your calendar for close to a year, and if your due date is approaching, the flood of texts and calls to check in has probably already begun. Unfortunately, unless you have an induction or C-section scheduled, there is little chance that day will be his actual birthday, as (reminder!) only 5 percent of spontaneous vaginal births actually happen on the projected due date.[3] Sixty-six percent occur within seven days, but it turns out the way we calculate gestational age just isn't very precise.

That's why it's best to look at your due date as a guess or range, not a guarantee. The majority of practitioners stick with dating from your last menstrual period, but not everyone ovulates on cycle day fourteen, not all cycles are twenty-eight days, and not every embryo docks in the uterus on the same schedule. There's also human error to factor in, as it's easy to forget or misreport your LMP. Another factor: genetics and family history. If your mother, sister, or mother-in-law had a particularly long pregnancy, so, too, could you.[4]

But what about those third-trimester ultrasound measurements (if you had them)? Wouldn't those be more exact? We touched on this before, but it turns out no. In the first months of pregnancy, babies are about the same size regardless of how large they will grow to be at birth, which is why they map pretty closely to LMP. In the final months, measurements and dating are based on an average that just isn't accurate for some larger babies. Trying to estimate weight toward the end can also be surprisingly imprecise, and be off by one or two pounds.

For first-time mothers, the estimated due date may actually be three to five days after forty weeks,[5] and there is no difference in pregnancy duration based on the baby's gender. Fifty percent of first-time mothers will go into labor on their own by forty weeks and five days, and 75 percent will give birth by forty-one weeks and two days. If you are coordinating your birth and postpartum support, give them a date with a week on either end.

The last few weeks of pregnancy are an important developmental period for your baby, so though you may be ready to eject them from your uterus after such a long stay (and, of course, you're excited to meet them), don't rush too much. You can't put them back in once they come out.

### Into the breech

Some babies have a hard time finding the exit. About 3 to 4 percent of pregnancies end in what's known as a breech birth, where instead of arriving at the cervix headfirst, the baby arrives with butt or legs pointed down.[6] Attempting to give birth with a baby in the breech position is dangerous, and was a common cause of infant mortality in the days before modern medicine. Two of the top complications are cord prolapse (the cord comes out of the cervix before the baby) and the baby's head getting stuck (head entrapment). If breech presentation can't be fixed before birth, most physicians mandate a C-section. Few physicians are willing to attempt vaginal breech births, or are trained sufficiently, as the risks are high for you and your baby.

Breech babies are usually detected halfway through the third trimester, which provides time to try to turn them before they are full term. One low-risk but painful method to correct it is called external cephalic version (ECV). It's been around since the days of Aristotle, and has become increasingly popular in the US since the 1980s.

ECV involves manually turning the baby around at thirty-six or thirty-seven weeks. It always happens in a hospital just in case it causes premature labor. A doctor or midwife applies firm pressure and gently turns the baby up and away from the pelvis. Some women find it just slightly uncomfortable; others describe it as excruciating as labor, which is why an epidural is sometimes offered. ECV works in 60 to 75 percent of cases, and once the baby is pointed in the right direction, it has less than a 5 percent chance of going breech again before birth.[7] However, not everyone can try it. Carrying multiples, previous C-sections, low levels of amniotic fluid, placenta previa, and other pregnancy complications exclude you.

If you can't try ECV, you still have options. Holding yourself in certain positions can help, and there are a number of different fetal positioning methodologies that suggest different movements and exercises. Acupuncture and chiropractic care are two alternative avenues.

Playing music near the pelvis is yet another. And if you like water, spending time floating in a pool with your belly down might entice a baby to flip.

### Are we there yet?

Sorry, there is no way to coax a baby out of your belly before they're ready. However, there are ways to (possibly) speed things up if you are at or past your due date. While the medical evidence isn't particularly definitive, the below methods won't do any harm.

- **Go for a walk or climb stairs.** Hills and inclines are less painful if you have pressure in your back, as is walking on softer surfaces like grass or a track. Coupled with a little fresh air, the exercise may also help you be less stir-crazy in the final weeks.
- **Sex.** Not only are these last weeks your final opportunity for intimacy sans baby, the female orgasm does double duty and releases oxytocin, which is the main ingredient in Pitocin, the most common medication to induce labor. Semen is high in prostaglandins, which powers one of the cervical-ripening drugs also used during induction.
- **Nipple stimulation.** Before trying this route, run it by your practitioner, as it can be powerful, especially if you have a high-risk pregnancy. If they say yes, it's exactly what it sounds like and you can do it manually or with a breast pump.
- **Acupuncture or acupressure.** Research is limited, but one study[8] shows that women at full term who receive acupuncture are more likely to go into labor on their own, and less likely to have a C-section. The hypothesis is that it stimulates the uterus via hormonal changes or the nervous system.[9] Acupuncture is most

effective when your cervix is already at least partially open for business, so make sure you coordinate timing with your care provider.

- **Eat dates.** Preliminary studies[10] have shown that eating six to eight Deglet Noor or three to four Medjool dates daily starting in week thirty-six helped women have higher rates of spontaneous delivery, shorter labor, and less need for induction.[11] It's thought that they help ripen the cervix. More is not better, so don't eat a whole bag thinking it's going to start labor. Even if it doesn't work, dates are packed with fiber, which helps with constipation.
- **Membrane sweep.** You'll need some help for this one. Also known as membrane stripping or a cervical sweep, it can bring on labor if you are nearing an induction or late. Your provider will put a finger into your cervix and with a circular motion separate the amniotic sac from the cervix and stimulate prostaglandins. It can be uncomfortable and cause spotting, and there is a risk of a ruptured amniotic sac. You may go into labor within hours afterward, or it may be that nothing happens.

The siren song of Internet ads or products promising a "natural" way to induce labor can be very tempting. But beware, as some products can actually do harm. Before using any teas, oils, or herbs claiming results, talk to your practitioner about the side effects.

*When forty weeks came and went with no action, I took long wad-dles to the park, marched up and down the stairs, used an electric pump to stimulate my nipples, had giant pregnant sex, doubled my date consumption, tried electrified acupuncture, and had two*

: *different membrane sweeps. Retrospectively, the membrane sweep* :
: *might be the one thing I'd skip if I had it to do over.* :

## Induction

Labor induction can happen for a variety of reasons: preeclampsia, gestational diabetes, premature rupture of membranes (your water broke but no labor is happening), not enough amniotic fluid, chorio-amnionitis (a uterine infection), and other medical conditions. The most common reason it's done is if pregnancies last beyond the due date.

If you hit the forty-two-week mark, the placenta may not be able to support the nutritional needs of your baby, and there is an increased risk of stillbirth. This is why most ob-gyns encourage induction at forty-one weeks if labor hasn't started on its own.[12] The ARRIVE study[13] (A Randomized Trial of Induction Versus Expectant Management) advocates induction at thirty-nine weeks, as it showed that healthy women who were electively induced between thirty-nine weeks and thirty-nine weeks, four days, were less likely to need a C-section. It is not standard protocol, but if you are seeing an ob-gyn, they may ask if you're interested. Most physicians still recommend letting nature take its course unless there is a compelling reason not to.

Seventy-five percent of first-time mothers who are induced go on to have a successful vaginal delivery, which means one in four still end up with a C-section.[14] The main factor that dictates the success or failure of an induction is how ripe your cervix is, and depending how far along things are, you can experience one of several induction routes.

The first is to ripen your cervix using prostaglandins or a Foley or bulb catheter. The Foley is a small balloon that is gradually inflated to dilate the cervix manually. Another method is an amniotomy, which involves physically rupturing the amniotic sac with a small hook. This is done only if the baby is well positioned and the cervix is at least partially dilated and effaced. The most well-known induction tool is Pitocin, a synthetic version of oxytocin, the hormone that causes the uterus to contract. Pitocin is not used to ripen the cervix, so you won't receive it until things are a bit further along. It usually makes labor contractions more intense, and can shorten the breaks between.

Induction does have risks. Oxytocin and prostaglandins can over-stimulate the uterus, decreasing blood flow through the placenta, which can then lower your baby's heart rate. The powerful contractions can also rupture scars from a prior C-section or other uterine surgery. And there can be more bleeding after delivery, as sometimes your uterine muscles get fatigued and then don't contract when you need them to. Most OBs won't suggest it if you have placenta previa, a breech baby, umbilical cord prolapse, active genital herpes, or any other condition that would be unsafe for the two of you.

### *Early signs of labor*

The insane truth is, we have no idea exactly what triggers labor. One widely discussed hypothesis is that babies are born right before they will no longer be able to navigate the narrow human pelvis on the way out, or that a chemical produced in the baby's lungs alerts the mother that they are now capable of breathing on their own. Yet another is that the length of a pregnancy is limited by the mother's metabolism. Whatever the trigger, and hopefully science will put some muscle behind finding the answer, there are well-established symptoms that tell you labor is imminent.

### Braxton Hicks contractions

You may have been feeling these practice contractions throughout the third trimester, but closer to birth the frequency will increase. So how do you tell the difference? Braxton Hicks, known as false labor, will cause your uterus to harden, but moving or changing positions often makes them stop. Real contractions are like a moving train.

They don't stop, and get more intense and frequent over time. True labor is often so painful that you will be rendered speechless.

### Baby drops

For first-time moms, the baby drops farther into the pelvis two to four weeks before labor starts. "Lightening," as it is also called, can also happen at the start of labor. The good news: Breathing will be easier now that your baby isn't pressing on your lungs. The bad news: Your baby will now be exerting pressure on your bladder, which will multiply your round trips to the bathroom.

### Cervical ch-ch-changes

Think of your cervix like a turtleneck. It stretches and thins to accommodate the baby during birth, then returns to its original size. Cervical changes are key to birth, and one of the first signs of labor your practitioner will look for is cervical dilation, or opening. It begins at one centimeter and, by the time your baby's head is peeking out, will grow to ten centimeters.

But birth is not just about cervical dilation. In order for your baby to exit successfully, cervical dilation *and* effacement need to happen. Cervical effacement, or ripening, is the thinning of the cervix. During labor, your cervix shortens and pulls up and actually becomes part of the uterine wall. Effacement is measured as a percentage, and, like dilation, can also happen slowly in the weeks before labor, or more suddenly during labor itself.

### Diarrhea

Though your stomach may get squirrelly anytime during pregnancy, diarrhea is more likely to happen in the weeks and days before labor starts. Why? Because of chemicals called prostaglandins and because, alas, your rectum, like the muscles in the rest of your body, is relaxing to prepare for birth. Keep a bathroom within easy waddling distance.

## Weight loss or stabilization

The increase in bathroom breaks coupled with the lower levels of amniotic fluid may mean your weight gain stops, and that you even drop a few pounds in the final weeks of your pregnancy. Have no fear—this has nothing to do with your baby's health.

## Bloody show and mucus plug

Though it sounds more like a horror movie, the appearance of the bloody show and mucus plug are happy signs you'll meet your baby soon. The opening of your cervix is blocked throughout pregnancy by a mucus plug, designed to keep bacteria and other bad stuff out. But imagine draining a bathtub: When your baby is ready to make their appearance, the plug will come out, pre-labor, accompanied by thick discharge. Spotting is normal, but if you experience heavy bleeding, call your practitioner immediately. There is no need to store and carry your mucus plug to labor and delivery or text a picture of it to your practitioner. They've seen hundreds, and unless there is something really weird happening, they all kind of look the same.

## Water breaks

While rom-coms would have you believe that it happens as a gush in the produce section, usually your water breaking is much less dramatic. Sometimes it's a trickle of amniotic fluid. Occasionally, it's a very watery surprise. Other times, it's hard to even notice and happens in the middle of the night as you're sleeping.

When it happens, your first move should be to call your practitioner as you are officially in labor. There is, however, one exception. In 8 to 10 percent of pregnancies, water breaks before labor without contractions. This is called premature rupture of the membranes (PROM) and may mean an induction is imminent.[15] Why? Because a ruptured amniotic sac is at risk for infection if labor takes too long to start.

If you feel that whoosh and it's green or brown, that could mean meconium (your baby's first bowel movement) in the amniotic fluid, which can be dangerous if swallowed. Bright red is another sign you should see someone immediately.

## THE STAGES OF LABOR

### *Stage 1*

### Early labor

Early labor is the longest and mildest phase of labor. It can last anywhere from six to twenty-four hours (sometimes longer), and will get your cervix to three or four centimeters dilated. If you're wondering if you are actually in labor, just remember the phrase "longer, stronger, closer together" and apply it to your contractions. It's one way you can tell a contraction is the real thing versus Braxton Hicks. The other is that moving around or drinking water won't make contractions go away—they will remain intense for thirty to forty-five seconds.

Since it takes a while to kick into active labor, and most hospitals will not admit you until you are in it, it's time to get comfortable at home. Distractions designed to keep you relaxed and your anxiety at a minimum are key during these early hours. Achy back? A warm shower or heating pad is a great solution. Most physicians suggest avoiding the tub after your bag breaks to avoid infection, so if you can wait for your warm bath until you get to the hospital, that's best.

Though it may seem unavoidable, don't forget to pee. A full bladder can slow labor from progressing. If you're hungry, now is not the time to scarf down a pizza. Have a light snack. Once contractions are less than five minutes apart, it's go to the hospital or birth center time.

Now to the inevitable question: What does labor pain feel like? It is categorized in two ways: visceral pain and somatic pain.[16]

Visceral pain comes during the initial stages of labor and is described as internal pain—dull or aching, squeezing, and sometimes sickening, as it can be accompanied by nausea and vomiting. It can feel vague and diffuse, as it's not typically confined to one area. During phase one of labor, the uterus pushes the baby against the cervix so it dilates in order to move him through the vagina. Most women compare it to really intense menstrual cramps.

Somatic pain comes once the vagina stretches and opens, beginning late in early labor and continuing through active labor. It is much more intense, localized, and easier to pinpoint, and is described as a sharp or burning feeling as the pelvic floor, perineum, and vagina stretch and distend, and uterine contractions intensify.

If your next question is *When will I know when it's time to leave the house?*, the answer is in that phrase "longer, stronger, closer together." You should have a strong contraction lasting one minute every four to five minutes for at least an hour before you bolt. If you can talk through the contraction, it's probably not strong enough.

## Active labor

Congratulations, your cervix graduated from three centimeters dilated and will soon be closer to seven. Active labor takes an average of eight hours, but could take up to eighteen. Oof. By now you'll likely be in the hospital or birthing center (if you're not, it's time to go!), and whoever is there to coach and support you will be fully engaged.

Your attention will likely be focused on the rise and fall of contractions by now, so if you haven't already, pull out the labor coping and relaxation methods you've been practicing so you can preserve your energy and try to stay calm. If you did not get an epidural, walking around or trying different positions or a warm bath is a good distraction. If you're in the thick of it and feel like you need more pain management, now is a good time to ask for that, too. Get some rest before the final stage (if you can).

The use of perineal warm packs during this stage of labor can prevent third- and fourth-degree tearing, and reduce the instances of urinary incontinence at twelve months.[17] If you are working with a doula, this is something she may do. If not, nurses and partners are good candidates for this job.

### Transitional labor

So named because it is a transition from labor to pushing, transitional labor is the shortest and most challenging phase, taking between thirty minutes and four hours. Your cervix dilates from seven centimeters to ten, and contractions will last between one and two minutes with a thirty-second to two-minute rest between.

Transitional labor is tough, so lean on your support person as much as you can—literally and figuratively. It's not always pretty, either. Symptoms you may run into include chills and hot flashes, nausea and vomiting, and other forms of gastric distress.

## Stage 2

### Pushing

Fire up the hip-hop—it's time to push it. Your cervix is fully dilated at ten centimeters, and you will start to feel an intense urge to push. The pushing phase can last from twenty minutes to three hours, depending on how the baby is positioned. Contractions will be forty-five to ninety seconds, with three to five minutes of rest in between. Take every moment of rest you can, and use a mirror to check things out if you need extra encouragement, or are just curious.

The best part of this phase is that it ends with the first glimpse of your baby's head crowning. That feeling, while magical, can also involve a lot of burning or stinging (there's a reason the crowning effect earned it the nickname "the ring of fire"), as your vagina and perineum are stretching to their limits. When the baby starts crowning, your provider may tell you not to push anymore. Controlling the rate of the head crowning is how your ob-gyn or midwife prevents tears. Warning, if you're using a mirror to monitor progress, the head can slip in and out. It doesn't mean you are stalling—just stay focused and listen to your coaches.

There may be poop. Yes, the rumors are true—though it doesn't happen to everyone, many women pee and/or poop during this phase of birth. Mentally prepare yourself and your partner that it's not only normal but common, and one of the many reasons the beds in labor and delivery rooms have waterproof covers. The medical staff is well equipped to do a cleanup, so you won't be sitting in anything unsavory for long.

After your baby's head has fully emerged, they will turn one last time to face your side and slip their shoulders out. And the rest of their body will follow.

Finally, the nine long months are OVER!

Oh, wait. Sorry. One last thing.

## Stage 3

### Delivering the placenta

Though it would be nice to hang the "mission accomplished" banner and leave the world behind to enjoy uninterrupted snuggles with your newborn, if you deliver vaginally, there is one final step before you are truly done with birth: delivering the placenta, or as it's also known, the afterbirth.

The placenta, the magical organ that grew to nourish and take care of your baby during pregnancy, is no longer necessary. Usually it comes out between five and thirty minutes following birth, and sometimes in the emotional rush of seeing your baby for the first time, you may not notice it's happening. You'll experience mild contractions (especially in comparison to what was going on earlier!) that help move the placenta through the birth canal, and your midwife or doctor may apply pressure to your uterus or even pull lightly on the cord to speed things along. Sometimes they will also administer a shot of oxytocin that helps minimize postpartum bleeding, shrinks the uterus, and helps expel the placenta. Once the placenta is out, it will be examined, and if it is intact, you're back to bonding time with the baby.

## CESAREAN SECTIONS

C-sections, or belly births, are the most common major surgical procedure performed today. The World Health Organization pegs the ideal cesarean section rate at 10 percent, but in the US, it's over 30 percent and climbing.

C-sections can be prescheduled due to medical conditions or obstetrical complications, like a breech baby, or in the case of multiples. They can also happen unexpectedly during vaginal deliveries if the cord becomes tangled, in cases of placental abruption or previa (when the placenta is covering part or all of the cervix), if labor stops progressing, and in cases of uterine rupture, a baby in distress, a baby too large for the pelvis, or labor stalling out. For sufferers of sexual assault or abuse, C-sections can reduce associations with trauma. However, because they are so common, there is a perception that they pose fewer risks and involve less pain than delivering vaginally, leading some women to want to schedule them without any medical need.

The phrase "too Posh to push" was inspired by Victoria Beckham's decision to schedule her C-section. Though she later claimed it was for a medical condition, the main reasons cited in the case of scheduled C-sections are convenience and control over the timing of birth, anxiety related to labor pain, and fear of urinary incontinence and stretching. While the idea of not laboring for hours or days is, let's be honest, appealing, if you're thinking about it for these reasons, there are considerations to weigh. Not to mention your doctor may not even allow C-sections on maternal request.

C-sections are major abdominal surgery. Your hospital stay will be two to three days—twice that of a vaginal birth—and at-home recovery is typically several weeks longer. Planned C-sections are associated with increased risk of postpartum complications and infection versus vaginal delivery, and present a higher risk of maternal death[18] and of uterine rupture in future pregnancies. You will also be left with an abdominal scar, which generally can be covered by your underwear or bathing suit but will take time to heal. If you're trying to avoid incontinence, studies have shown that in some cases you are just as likely to suffer from it as you would after a vaginal birth, and that at best, the rate is just 8.4 percent lower.[19]

Babies born via C-section have less beneficial gut bacteria[20] and are more likely to develop allergies and asthma. If you plan to breastfeed, a C-section also increases the time until you can initiate your first session, and often delays milk coming in by several days. Delivering before thirty-nine weeks, which is the recommended timeline for a scheduled C-section, can also lead to developmental delays and may mean time in the NICU.

If your practitioner recommends prescheduling a C-section, or suggests it during a long labor, make sure they explain why. One of the unfortunate realities of today's medical system is the indirect financial incentives that can influence the type of care you receive. For example, doctors and hospitals are paid more for C-sections,[21] which can bias them in that direction, especially in cases where labor is taking forever. There is also liability to consider,[22] as medical malpractice lawsuits related to complications for mothers are much easier and cheaper to defend than those related to the lives of babies.

Ultimately, the decision should be made after a discussion weighing the pros and cons with your physician, as there are certainly situations where a C-section is more beneficial than vaginal birth.[23] And if you do decide it's the best way, or if a medical reason pops up during a planned vaginal delivery, getting a C-section doesn't mean you will be any less of a parent or failed a test. The goal is a healthy baby and a healthy mom. C-sections are often necessary to make that happen.

### *What to expect during a C-section*

How it starts is dependent on what led you to a C-section. If it was planned, the whole experience is pretty chill. If it's an emergency, it will be less so. The whole surgery usually takes between forty-five minutes and one hour from start to finish.

If you haven't already received an epidural or IV, one will be inserted to numb your lower body and allow for the delivery of other medications. Next, you'll be moved to the operating room, where the doctors will set up the surgical field and clean your stomach. There will be a curtain draped between you and where they cut, though many hospitals now provide the option of a "gentle C-section," which means the curtain is dropped so you can actually see your baby as they are lifted out.

Today's C-section incisions are usually discreet, and around four to six inches long. Most cuts are horizontal and happen below your bikini line (hence why they are also known as bikini cuts). Vertical cuts are used only when the baby is premature or in a difficult position, or the mother is obese. The first cut opens your skin, the second cuts through your fascia, and the third goes into your uterus. The baby is then lifted out. If everything is okay, your partner can cut the umbilical cord and you can try breastfeeding or have skin-to-skin time. The placenta will be removed after the cord is cut, and the last step is to stitch you up.

So what does it feel like? Answer: not much. Once the epidural or spinal block kicks in, the only sensations are pressure and tugging, as the ob-gyn pushes on your abdomen to help deliver your baby, and sometimes cold from the freezing OR and medications. Nausea is another common side effect, and can happen during or after the surgery.

## WHAT HAPPENS RIGHT AFTER BIRTH

Sometimes called the "golden hour," those first sixty minutes are your first opportunity to bond, try out breastfeeding if that's your plan, and enjoy that new-baby smell. The first physical assessments of your baby can actually be done while they are resting on your chest, and all the weighing, measuring, bathing, and other medical procedures can wait until after those first sixty minutes.

### Events for baby

Your baby just entered the world, and it's already time for their first exams. When and whether they receive some of them is up to you, and something you put into your birth preferences. But it's important to understand what to expect, and to address any areas of strong preference with your care team before they're in the middle of it post-birth.

### Apgar test

The Apgar test is typically given one and five minutes after birth to see if your baby needs any extra care. Named for its inventor, Dr. Virginia Apgar, it grades babies in five areas:

- Appearance (skin color—from bluish to good color)
- Pulse (heart rate—from zero to more than 100 beats/ minute)
- Grimace (reflex irritability—from no reaction to being pinched to a cough or cry)
- Activity (muscle tone—from limp to active)
- Respiration (breathing effort—from no cry to strong cry)

Each category is worth two points, for a maximum Apgar score of ten. Babies who score a seven or more are considered very healthy. Perfectly healthy babies can have low Apgar scores at the minute mark, but 98 percent of babies reach a score of seven after five minutes out of the womb.

### *Cord clamping*

The American College of Obstetricians and Gynecologists endorses[24] delayed cord clamping to allow more blood to flow to your baby's body in the first minutes after birth. This means instead of immediately cutting the cord when your baby arrives, there will be a pause until it stops pulsing.

### *Heel-stick test*

Before you and your new addition leave the hospital, a few drops of your baby's blood is collected from their heel, in a procedure appropriately known as the heel-stick test. It screens for heritable and genetic conditions, and is typically paid for by insurance. It's done early in life because many heritable conditions can be treated before they cause any serious health problems.

Every state's public health department mandates screens for different conditions after a hospital birth, so if you'd like specifics, you can visit www.babysfirsttest.org to see what is offered in your area. Tests vary due to costs and laws, frequency of specific disorders in certain states, availability of treatments for each condition, and funding sources. Typically, you'll receive the results from your pediatrician a few weeks later.

### *Eye drops, vitamin K shot, bathing, circumcision*

The birth preferences you put together should address all of his. But as a reminder, there is a standard course of care that all infants born in hospitals receive. When and whether they receive some of them is up to you, so address this in the early stages of labor so your care team knows your preferences ahead of time.

Eye drops and the vitamin K shot are typically administered an hour after birth. The first bath is optional, and can be delayed until you go home. If you give birth in a hospital, circumcision (if requested) usually happens within forty-eight hours of birth. Sometimes the procedure happens later in a pediatrician's office or is performed a few weeks later, especially if it's done for religious reasons.

### Hearing test

Ninety-eight percent of all newborns receive this screening.[25] Babies with hearing challenges require special care. Early interventions can improve their development, communication, and language abilities. It is quick and painless, and can be done while they are sleeping.

There are two methods to screen newborn hearing. The first uses headphones to play tones and clicks, and electrodes on the baby's head measure their brain response. The second method measures the response when clicks are played into the baby's ears through a tiny probe in their ear canal.

### Congenital heart defect screening

The critical congenital heart defect (CCHD) test looks for low oxygen levels, which can indicate issues with your baby's heart. This is another noninvasive, painless screening that happens twenty-four hours after birth. A small sensor will be attached to your baby's skin, then attached to an oximeter, which measures their oxygen levels.

Around 7,200 babies per year are born with critical CHDs,[26] and may need surgery or help in the first year of life.

## THE POSTPARTUM STAY

In the case of a C-section, once you're stitched up, you'll be wheeled into a recovery room, then into your postpartum room for a few nights of observation. After a vaginal birth, you may receive stitches to repair any tears in your vagina and/or perineum, which can be quite painful. Expect a two-to-three-night stay after a C-section, and one or two nights for a vaginal birth.

If you plan to breastfeed, your baby will room in with you, or be brought in from the nursery every few hours. Don't beat yourself up if things are not working immediately. We'll get into this in greater detail later, but your milk can take time to come in—especially after a C-section—so if you need to supplement with formula or require assistance with breastfeeding, that's not only okay, it's normal.

*Now that you've read what the textbooks say about childbirth, you may wonder how mine went. Even though I was an overprepared person penning a book about pregnancy who researched and understood every possible birth scenario, mine was a prime example of things not going at all according to plan.*

*Based on his activity level, and the nonstop kicks in the ribs, I assumed our son would spring into the world on time, or even early. But as we approached forty-one weeks, at which point I was giant and impatient, he was still comfortably nestled in my abdomen, hiccuping away.*

*Forty-one weeks is generally the cutoff for induction, especially if you are of advanced maternal age. Knowing what I know about due date accuracy, I chose to give him a few more days to emerge voluntarily before any intervention. The induction was scheduled for forty-one weeks, three days, so two days before, I went in for a final fetal monitoring session and amniotic fluid measurement. The medical team suggested a second membrane sweep to encourage some action. Later that night, I woke up thinking I had wet the bed. No rom-com-style public gush for me—my water broke while I was sleeping.*

*Hours of trickle-trickle-trickle later (and a few text sessions with our doulas) and we knew it was time. We spent the day waiting for something to happen, and though I was uncomfortable, the contractions were not dramatic enough to constitute active labor. This was unfortunate, because when your amniotic sac breaks, active labor needs to start quickly, or the risk of infection goes up. Knowing we should report to the hospital that evening, I saw my cozy plan for active labor at home with Nick, our dog, and our doulas slip away. So after one last dinner, we loaded up our go bags and drove to the hospital.*

*There was no wait in triage for us; we went straight into a labor and delivery room, likely because my bag had already been open for almost twenty-four hours, and I was technically well past my due date. The first doctor urged an immediate Pitocin hookup to jump-start labor, but I demanded my full twenty-four hours (and a few critical hours of sleep) to see if things would start on their own. Thank goodness we did, because I needed rest for the adventure ahead.*

*The little guy still refused to budge, so at one to two centimeters dilated, I started on Pitocin early the next morning, with the dosage increasing every thirty minutes. Over a sandwich and rice krispies treat with my best friend a few hours later, the contractions came on strong and suddenly, along with intense nausea.*

*I chose not to get an epidural, so I wasn't confined to bed and could have an active labor. Instead, nitrous and the comfort measures we had practiced, like breathing, the TENS machine, and soaks in the tub, were my coping mechanisms. Even with Nick and our doulas as full-time coaches, the help of a midwife and labor nurse, and the nitrous mask, my memory of the ten hours I spent moving between the tub and bed and birthing stool and yoga ball is a complete blur. Though I was well trained, eventually I coped by yelling into the nitrous mask at the height of contractions (not recommended) and squeezing a small plastic comb in my hand like Dumbo and his magic feather as a distraction.*

*I've never been a particularly modest person, and after all the pregnancy exams I doubted I had any modesty left.*

*But labor really put a nail in it. I started the day optimistically, in my own cute hospital gown brought from home, but after my first trip to the tub, I was fully and unapologetically naked for the rest of it. Nudity isn't mandatory, of course, but if you're planning tub time during labor, it's probably how you'll end up.*

*Pitocin intensifies contractions, and unfortunately for me, mine were very close together. I had only thirty seconds of ebb between each to chill versus the typical two to three minutes. Channeling my breath and sending the energy down to my cervix, the way I'd practiced, went straight out the window as the pain sharpened.*

*Labor pain is hard to articulate. Friends described it as the worst menstrual cramps of their lives. My lower back, which felt alternately like an elephant was using it as a stool and my spine was ripping in half, was the main issue. Time in the tub helped, but it was still excruciating. I found out later that I was actually in back labor, as my son had turned and was stuck facing the wrong way.*

*One benefit of vaginal birth with no epidural is that I could feel the little guy making the trip down my pelvis toward the exit. At times, I even felt an urge to push. However, around 8 p.m., the movement ground to a halt. I noted the time and gave myself another hour to see if anything would change, but mentally started to prepare for yet another unexpected twist.*

*After discussing the options with Nick and our doula, we decided it was time to see if an epidural would help things relax and open. My suspicion was that his massive head was stuck, so for the first time, I acknowledged to myself that a C-section might be required. If that happened, an epidural would be necessary anyway, so it seemed like the right move.*

*The decision was cemented after the most frustrating cer-*

*vical exam of my life. After ten hours of intense labor and Pitocin, I was still only four centimeters dilated, and not fully effaced. The amniotic sac had been open for almost forty-eight hours, which meant infection was increasingly possible.*

*The astounding pain relief from the epidural melted those concerns away temporarily. I was bummed not to be able to get out of bed, but after such a long day, it was a very welcome break. On went the hospital gown, up went the Pitocin, and in went the Foley catheter (a tube that goes into the bladder to drain urine), which oddly didn't work even after it was inserted a second time.*

*After a somewhat restful night, the Pitocin was nearly maxed out, and I was still only five centimeters dilated and not fully effaced. Apparently, my cervix also had a lip that was blocking his progress. And there was more bad news. My white blood cell count was elevated, which meant chorioamnionitis, an infection in my uterus. My creatinine levels were also high, indicating my kidneys were no longer doing their job. And the catheter still wasn't working twelve hours later. The combination of symptoms led the team to conclude I had preeclampsia with severe features, which meant a magnesium sulfate drip to avoid progression to eclampsia. I knew that condition as the one that killed Sybil in Downton Abbey, so we agreed to the treatment.*

*Knowing the goal was a vaginal birth, the medical team gave us a few more hours before we had to talk plan B. Gambling with my health for a little longer was fine. But the minute little dude showed any distress, it was game over.*

*When we hit the deadline, I was only at six centimeters, my bag had been open for over sixty hours, and his heart rate started to spike. As soon as that happened, I called it. No more interventions—it was time to get him out.*

*Watching the medical team mobilize for the C-section was the first time I felt like a patient in a medical procedural. Within fifteen minutes I was wheeled into an overly bright operating room, surrounded by what seemed like dozens of doctors, and lifted onto a skinny bed. The drape was raised, more pain management hit, Nick and our doula sat by my side, and the procedure began. Though I was pretty alert considering the sheer volume of pharmaceuticals coursing through my body, my focus was less on whatever they were doing to me and more on our labor playlist, which we brought into the OR. Mixed with the whoosh that I later found out was compressed air to create space in my abdomen, the music was a perfect distraction from the light pressure I felt as they tried to fish the baby out.*

*Then, the sound every new parent dreams about: our baby's first cry. Hearing his scream of outrage after being wrenched unwillingly from my body was perhaps the most remarkable moment of my life. And even more surreal—he was no longer an abstract bump. He was a tiny human with lungs and vocal cords that Nick and I had made.*

*The drape was dropped, and for the first time, we saw our beautiful little boy. And he had quite the cone head after so much time wedged in my pelvis. We later found out his head was stuck and crushing my ureter, hence why I hadn't peed in nearly eighteen hours. It also meant the preeclampsia diagnosis was incorrect, and that the magnesium drip that caused excessive bleeding during surgery was in fact unnecessary.*

*After a quick check of his vitals, Nick cut the cord and they brought him over to me. The medications stirred up some serious nausea, so it wasn't the perfect skin-to-skin session I'd envisioned. But the relief that he was out and healthy trumped any disappointment felt in how it ended.*

*In the anemic weeks recovering from the C-section, I thought about what we could have done differently. I replayed the experience with Nick and our doulas and asked them the same question. We all agreed we might go back and skip the membrane sweep, but probably would have ended up in the same spot, as my pelvis wasn't wide enough to accommodate his giant head (though I maintain that my vagina \*is\* HUGE!!!).*

*Failure to progress and overreaction to jumps on the fetal monitor are two areas that medicine, frankly, doesn't fully understand. Further research on these subjects could help reduce the rate of unnecessary C-sections. Knowing this gave me pause. But in our situation, given the three liters of fluid locked up in my bladder with no escape path and spikes on my labs, I couldn't afford to be inflexible about sticking to vaginal birth at any cost.*

*I did every bit of research possible (hell, I wrote the sections on birth right before it happened) and planned for the experience that I wanted. And I'll admit it: I thought none of this would happen to me because I was so well prepared. But just goes to show that it can happen to anyone.*

*Did I want a vaginal birth? Yes. And I endured over sixty hours of labor and every possible route to make that happen. In the days before C-sections, I probably would have died during childbirth. My pelvis just isn't big enough to accommodate a baby's head, much less a large baby like my eight-pound-five-ounce son's. So thank God for modern medicine.*

# THIRD-TRIMESTER CHECKLIST

☐   Attend birth class (breastfeeding and infant CPR are also worth looking into).

☐   Take a tour of your chosen hospital or center before birth.

☐   Talk to work about the final details of your maternity leave.

☐   Apply to add your baby to insurance (this can also be done after birth, depending on your policy).

☐   Choose a pediatrician.

☐   Preregister for your hospital or birth center stay.

☐   Book your six-week (or sooner!) postpartum visit, which you can project using your due date.

☐   Pack your hospital bag (don't forget partner and baby!).

☐   Prep the nursery (wash clothes and blankets so everything is ready).

☐   Finalize post-birth support and back-to-work childcare.

☐   Take a few maternity photos (professionals not required— your friend or partner can play photographer).

☐   Set aside time to take care of yourself (pedicure, yoga, face mask—whatever makes you feel pampered and good).

☐   Plan post-birth meals (freeze meals, and let friends and family help).

☐   Schedule a last pre-baby date night with your partner.

☐   Install your car seat (can't leave the hospital without it!).

☐   Stock up on postpartum items.

# The Fourth Trimester

t's all over! You're no longer pregnant, and have a brand-new baby in your arms. Mission: Accomplished. Right?

Wrong!

Back in the days of multigenerational households, there was more exposure to pregnancy and its aftermath. But in today's nuclear families, much of our collective perspective comes from polished narratives on social media. So in the spirit of continued honesty and not avoiding the hard parts, here is a sneak peek into what life is like in the fourth trimester.

Your body will be a constipated, deflated, leaking hot mess of hormones, oddly colored discharge, and milk in those first weeks after birth. You will be sleep deprived. Your mind will be fuzzy. The hormonal surges won't stop even though the baby exited your body. And the mental transition from pregnant to parent is huge. Most new parents, if they're candid, will admit that they had to throw their expectations out the window and just go with the flow.

Some parents immediately feel a swell of indescribable love for their baby at birth. But if it takes a while for you to bond, there's nothing wrong. Infants emerge helpless, without the ability to clearly communicate their needs, and there is a lot of guesswork before you figure them out. You'd think the nine months of bodily cohabitation mean you already know each other well, but every baby has a set of opinions, preferences, and personality all their own. Some are predictable in utero, others less so. And your ability to mold and shape this new tiny human will be limited by who they are when they pop out.

During your stay in the postpartum wing, you'll be surrounded by nurses, lactation consultants, pediatricians, and OBs who will check in, help swaddle or put the baby to sleep, and dispense as much or as little advice as you'd like. At some point, you and your partner will find yourselves discharged and standing on the hospital curb with your brand-new human, thinking, *Now what?*

If you thought there were strong opinions about how to manage your pregnancy the "right way," just wait for the pressure related to breastfeeding, shedding your pregnancy weight, and managing baby-related accessories and routines when you get home. The mom-on-mom judgment is ruthless, and in many ways the hardest criticism to handle, since it's so unexpected.

Knowing all of this, be open to help. Remember what the word *partner* actually means, and find ways to let yours pitch in, whether it's just holding the baby for a while, doing some feedings, taking over chores, or keeping you company while you're trapped on the couch. For friends and family who offer assistance, let them provide meals and do laundry. Prefer not to have visitors? There are delivery services that can also reduce your long list of to-dos.

As with the rest of this book, the majority of this section is about you and your recovery. However, since baby isn't a native language for most new parents, we'll also explore their basic behaviors to help you decipher—and hopefully reduce—the tears.

*After my C-section, it was off to the recovery room for a few hours. Mr. Baby (a nickname my son earned for looking like a full-grown man straight out of the womb, and for his adult-volume burps) was plunked into my arms. I had no clue what I was doing, where I was, or what was going to happen next.*

*I was out of bed that first afternoon. By day two, I could slowly shuffle around the ward with Nick, who was pushing Mr. Baby in his wheeled crib. Our stay was a total of five nights, so the occasional stroll was definitely called for. A friendly warning: Don't get too close to any of the exits with your baby. After birth, babies are tagged with an ankle sen-*

*sor designed to go off if anyone tries to leave the postpartum ward with them. Proximity to the doors will trigger the baby-snatcher alarm, which blasts floor-wide. Very, very loudly. This advice definitely **not** given from firsthand experience of setting them off.*

*Disrupting the postpartum unit aside, there was also the practical side of my recovery. To have the privilege of catheter removal, you must pee a certain amount on your own, or it goes right back in. My plumbing was off, courtesy of Mr. Baby's head crushing my ureter, so it took a few tries before I could be disconnected. In the meantime, I carried the bag of urine around like a chihuahua in a Chanel. It was not, however, a convenient accessory when I was ready for a shower. With my little pet, an IV hookup, and a chair to support me, it was both the most logistics-heavy shower I've ever taken (where does one hang a bag of urine in a hospital shower?) and also possibly the GOAT. For me, there was nothing more life-affirming than rinsing it all off, especially since I had my own toiletries and towels from home. The cherry on top: finally sliding into my own clothes.*

*The "now what?" moment didn't hit until we were discharged and had arrived home. We thought we had everything we needed for those early days. But, as with birth, there were many things we didn't anticipate. Like Mr. Baby's Houdini-like ability to escape from every swaddle type but one, which is basically a baby straitjacket. How many wipes we would blow through cleaning poop that made it out of his diaper and up his back. Or how he was too long for newborn clothes after just days, and needed toddler-size socks for his hobbit-like feet at eight weeks.*

*Even with both sets of our parents visiting and amazing support, the first weeks home were a blur. My brain was different, my body was different, and life in general was unrecognizable. Not to mention we had a tiny, bellowing stranger around whose needs we didn't fully (or at all) understand.*

*Navigating stairs and getting in and out of bed were very uncomfortable. As with pregnancy, getting up with a C-section incision required a roll to the side, versus sitting up straight. That mistake was painful enough that I made it only once. My legs looked inflated, thanks to the many medications I was given during delivery. Compression leggings helped until the fluid and swelling disappeared later that week.*

*The only medications I took after my C-section were Tylenol and Motrin, on a rotating three-hour schedule. Surprisingly, the combo was effective, unless I got behind the pain. Managing the timing for all the different pills on top of infant feedings was impossible until I set alarm reminders on my phone.*

*And then there were the night sweats. My God. The drenching night sweats lasted for two weeks. It felt like waking up in a sauna. I kept a towel next to the bed or put one under me as I slept, or else the sheets would be soaked. The opposite happened when I visited the bathroom. Triggered by the fear that the effort would rip my sutures, I was hopelessly constipated. It took a combo of a laxative, a stool softener, and, finally, a suppository for me to get things moving. Trips there were not very productive (or too productive) for weeks. And rather than disappearing after pregnancy, my acid reflux actually intensified, making it hard to swallow.*

*In case you were wondering whether weighing yourself in the first six weeks is a good idea, I did it so you don't have to. The first day home, my weight was identical to the day I left for the hospital. Seventy-two hours of horrific night sweats later, it dropped twenty pounds. That's right—TWENTY POUNDS OF FLUID RETENTION LOST IN THREE DAYS. Seriously, postpartum weight fluctuations make no sense. Give your body time to recover, stop worrying that you'll never fit into your prepregnancy jeans, and STEP AWAY FROM THE SCALE.*

## SO WHAT'S HAPPENING OUT THERE?

### Month 1

**Baby:** Newborns have no sense of day and night, no schedule, and no idea that their arms and legs are attached to their body, since they do not yet understand what a body is! Their first days and weeks will mostly consist of sleeping, eating, soiling diapers, and crying. They can't see much or very far, and their lack of muscle makes them feel very fragile and floppy. Their eyes cross (when they're actually open), and there may be hiccups. But, man, do they smell good. Soak it in, as that delicious newborn fragrance doesn't last forever!

**You:** The first month after birth is pretty wild, so hang on tight. Your breasts will fill with milk, your hormones and emotions will ricochet up and down, and your former bump will shrink. The swelling and fluid retention vanish mostly in the form of sweating and peeing. Postpartum bleeding, known as lochia, will also include other random discharge, and lasts in some form for six to eight weeks. You might experience a touch (or a lot) of incontinence, as everything is stretched after pregnancy and birth. The baby blues or more serious depression can kick in, too, so if you are experiencing any downs, talk to someone you trust.

## Month 2

**Baby:** At the four- to six-week mark, your baby will be less lump-like and begin to do things like whip out a heart-melting smile. Cooing and gurgling can also start around now. The primary activities are still sleeping, eating, soiling diapers, and crying, though your baby will start to stay awake longer and be more interactive. It's a good time to introduce more visual stimuli (they love high-contrast, black-and-white images), or to test their grip using a rattle or other baby-safe toy. But warning: If they avoid eye contact or flap their arms wildly, you're in the overstimulation zone, and it's time for quiet.

**You:** Everyone's recovery after birth is different, and much of it depends on how your baby is eating and sleeping, and whether you are getting any rest. Bleeding should diminish, and if you aren't breastfeeding, the lochia may be replaced by your period. Yes, it can come back that fast. Ovulation can occur in the weeks even before your period returns, so if you are back in the saddle and having sex, use some form of birth control (unless you'd like to care for two children under the age of one). It's also time to get your pelvic floor back in shape, especially if you are experiencing any leaks or laxity. Your postpartum checkup happens this month, so plan to chat about any issues, physical or mental (and get birth control recommendations). One in five women reports depression during the first three months postpartum (and this number is assumed to be low), so if this is you, get the help you need.

## Month 3

**Baby:** Sleep is still the primary activity, but the time between naps will continue to increase, which means more time for play. The daily routine may take on a more consistent pattern, and goes something like: change diaper, feed, burp, play, nap, repeat. Every baby has a different internal clock, and everyone's parenting preferences are different, so find what works best for your family. Hands are the star attraction this month, and those tiny fists will be in your baby's mouth a lot. If you stick your baby in front of a mirror, they may not know it's their own reflection staring back, but it's entertaining to see them try to figure it out.

**You:** Postpartum hair loss can start around now, which means you may find larger-than-usual clumps of hair in your brush and shower. If your baby is sleeping for longer spans you may start to feel more rested; otherwise, the cumulative effects of sleep deprivation can be intense. Monitor your mental health, and make sure you have enough support. For many working moms, this is the last month at home. That alone can cause anxiety and stress. With that in mind, if you are breastfeeding and haven't begun pumping, you'll need to start, and introduce a bottle well in advance of your return to work.

## SYMPTOMS AND SOLUTIONS

While it's easy to assume that all of these issues are just part of the postpartum package, if something just doesn't feel right, you should call your care team instead of waiting until your checkup. This call is especially important if you are experiencing anxiety or depression, or physical issues like stress-induced incontinence, anal incontinence, instability in your pelvic floor, or excessive bleeding.

## Fourth-trimester symptoms and solutions

|  | When does it happen? | Symptoms |
|---|---|---|
| **Uterine contractions** | Mostly in the two to three days right after birth, especially while breastfeeding | Uncomfortable cramping and bleeding. It can be intense and feel like labor contractions. |
| **The baby blues** | May have started during pregnancy, but can kick into gear anytime after birth, most commonly in the first two weeks | Loss of interest in activities you used to love; decreased ability to feel pleasure; feelings of worthlessness, fear, or guilt, or suicidal thoughts |
| **Excessive sweating, especially as night sweats** | For the first weeks postpartum; peaks at two weeks, then tapers off | Waking up feeling like you just walked out of a steam room or shower, regardless of the temperature |
| **Hair loss** | Around three months postpartum. Will return to normal six to twelve months after birth, based on where you are in the growth cycle. | Finding more hair than usual in your shower and brush, sometimes in clumps |

| Cause | Solutions |
|---|---|
| Your uterus has to shrink from its watermelon size at birth back down to a fist, a process called involution. Breastfeeding stimulates the release of oxytocin, which in turn causes contractions. Your uterus will be back to its original size six weeks after birth, though this process can take longer with subsequent pregnancies. | Wait it out, unfortunately. Naproxen or ibuprofen are the most common medications, as they are allowed while breastfeeding.[1] Acetaminophen and aspirin come with side effects. A TENS machine can help you manage this pain. |
| Hormonal swings, physical shifts in your body, major life changes | Speak to your partner or someone else you trust, schedule an appointment with your doctor, contact a mental health professional, join a mom support group, or schedule a virtual appointment. |
| Your body's way of getting rid of the fluids you accumulated during pregnancy, triggered by low estrogen levels | Sleep on a towel (or keep one at the ready), drink more fluids, take a cool bath and go to bed with wet hair, and make sure your bedroom is a cool temperature. |
| Pregnancy and prenatal vitamins prevent hair from falling out at its normal rate. As soon as you give birth and your hormones drop, so too will your lush extra hairs. | Change up your shampoo and conditioner, try a different style or cut, use a volumizer, and keep taking that prenatal vitamin, especially if you are breastfeeding. |

## Fourth-trimester symptoms and solutions (continued)

| | When does it happen? | Symptoms |
|---|---|---|
| **Fatigue** | Forever? | Inability to keep your eyes open or form coherent sentences, generally feeling drained at all times |
| **Bleeding** | Heaviest in the first ten days after birth, it can last for four to six weeks. It also intensifies during and after breastfeeding as your uterus contracts. | Period-like bleeding that goes from red and pink to brown, and eventually yellow. If you see large clots, you fill a pad every hour, or there is a strong odor, call your provider. |
| **Perineal discomfort** | The exact time frame varies widely, but it is typically weeks or months after birth. | Varying degrees of specific pain if you had stitches, general discomfort, and numbness, made worse by coughing, sneezing, or laughing |
| **Incontinence (urine or poop)** | Can start during pregnancy, and goes days, weeks, months, or even years postpartum if not treated | Leaking urine, poop, or poop juice while laughing, sneezing, jumping, lifting, and running. Can also manifest as a sudden urge to pee outside of normal bathroom activities. |

| Cause | Solutions |
|-------|-----------|
| You gave birth and are now taking care of a newborn. Breastfeeding can also contribute, as it takes even more energy to produce milk. | Ask for help, go for a walk (seems counterintuitive, but it works!), employ all cheat codes such as food delivery and helpful friends, hydrate, sleep when the baby sleeps (even if just for a few minutes at a time). |
| Known as lochia, it's your body's way of getting rid of the extra blood, uterine tissue, and mucus left over from pregnancy. | No tampons allowed for six weeks after birth (whether it was vaginal or C-section), so once you run out of the hospital's mesh panties, it's pads for heavy days and period underwear or liners as things subside. Too much physical activity too soon will trigger increased bleeding, so take it easy. And opt for dark pants until it stops. |
| The stretching and pushing during birth, and the pressure of carrying a baby around for nine months. This pain isn't limited to vaginal births— you can also expect to have some discomfort with a C-section, especially if you labored first. | Start your pelvic floor exercises, sit on a donut (not the kind with sugar), pour or squirt water on the area with a peri bottle, use padsicles (recipe to follow), take a sitz bath, apply numbing agents, wear loose bottoms. |
| As with perineal discomfort, it's caused by the pressure the baby put on your pelvic floor during pregnancy, and stretching during birth. | Strengthening your pelvic floor with at-home exercises or seeing a pelvic floor therapist is step one. If you are experiencing fecal incontinence, have your anal tone checked by your ob-gyn. |

## Fourth-trimester symptoms and solutions (continued)

|  | When does it happen? | Symptoms |
|---|---|---|
| Trouble pooping | May be a sequel to pregnancy constipation, but can also start directly after birth and most commonly lasts for the first two weeks | Manifests as constipation and pain every time you try to go to the bathroom, or as the opposite problem—diarrhea and loose stool |
| Hemorrhoids | Might have started during pregnancy, and can last for months postpartum | Pain when you sit or go to the bathroom, itching, and bleeding |
| Nipple pain | Felt mostly during breastfeeding or while pumping | Tenderness or bleeding and cracking nipples, usually made worse during breastfeeding |
| Blocked ducts or mastitis | Any time while breastfeeding or pumping | Pain in breast tissue or a lump in the breast that is tender to the touch |

| Cause | Solutions |
|---|---|
| Post-birth pain medications make this worse, as can a sore perineum (the first poop after birth is kind of terrifying). | Eat fiber-packed foods (grains, fruit, roughage), drink plenty of fluids (you'll need it to make breast milk), take a walk. And if your provider offers stool softeners, say yes, please. |
| Swollen veins in your anus and lower rectum, caused by straining during pregnancy, birth, or trips to the bathroom | Eat a high-fiber diet, spot treat with witch hazel or tucks pads, stay hydrated, and try stool softeners. |
| A bad latch or bad positioning while breastfeeding, or vigorous sucking | Work on the underlying problem to avoid making it worse. Nipple butter and creams can help, along with cold compresses. Talk to a lactation consultant if it persists. |
| Can happen when a bra doesn't fit or is too tight, after engorgement, or if a nipple or duct is blocked | Massage your breast in the shower or use a warm compress before feedings. If you experience body aches and a fever over 100.4 degrees Fahrenheit along with the other symptoms, you may have an infection called mastitis, and should call your doctor immediately. You can get sepsis from untreated mastitis, so it's serious. |

## FOR PARTNERS

You watched your significant other go through pregnancy and child-birth (miraculous what the human body is capable of, right?), and now your job is to help her recover while transitioning to your own new identity as a parent. Don't forget about that communication practice you did during pregnancy. More than ever, it's important to check in with each other and keep an eye out for any signs she is struggling. Share responsibilities related to the baby, and give her space and time to take care of herself (and catch up on sleep!).

By the way, 10 percent of all new dads experience paternal post-partum depression,[2] so don't be surprised if you feel yourself strug-gling emotionally during this transition. Changes in household roles, financial concerns, new responsibilities, feelings about intimacy and sex, and return-to-work issues can all contribute. So if you need help, please get it.

### Role-playing

Sorry, this has a different meaning in a post-baby world (though, if done well and often, is still a massive turn-on — not that your partner is ready for sex right now!). You may already have a solid division of labor, and if so, you're ahead of most couples. If you don't, here are a few places to start:

- **Chief sanitation officer:** You change the diaper, she breastfeeds, you burp your new addition before he goes back to sleep.
- **Top chef:** Not a great cook? Now is a great time to learn easy recipes, the art of ordering in, or to say yes to that meal train from friends and family.
- **Vice president of errand running:** Gearing up a baby to go to the store can take longer, in the early days, than the whole round trip. Offer to do errands,

or if she wants to get out of the house, enjoy some time with the little one while she is gone.

Remember that there is a tremendous amount of pressure—external and self-imposed—on women to be perfect mothers and partners, while also performing at work and bouncing back physically. So don't wait for her to ask for help. Be proactive and offer up whatever assistance you can, as often as you can.

### Create some me-time (for her)

This may be something as simple as a hot bath or going for a walk alone or with a friend. She may not ask for it, and she may even turn you down the first few times you suggest it (mom guilt is real), but keep offering, and encourage her to do it. The huge benefit for you is that you will have solo bonding time with your baby—important, as you should be able to take over for your partner should an emergency arise. These early sessions can have a lasting and positive impact on your relationship with your baby, too.

### Help with breastfeeding and night feedings

Taking over one of the night feedings is perhaps the kindest way to help your partner start feeling like more of a human and less like a deflated zombie. Even if you can't do it in the first few weeks because she's exclusively breastfeeding, offer your company and help. Hanging out with a thirsty baby is tiring, repetitive, and, at times, lonely work. Bring her snacks or drinks, help her get more comfortable, wash bottles, burp the baby, or just keep her entertained.

### Become an early-parenting expert

During pregnancy, putting knowledge into practice was more about being empathetic and emotionally supportive for your partner. But now that your baby is here, you can take an equal role in the process of helping them learn and explore. Get to know the different stages of development, and build an environment to help their curious mind grow. And when one phase has passed, pack up the toys (and clothes they've outgrown!) for a friend or future child.

### Be patient in the bedroom

Sex after childbirth can take some time. The guidance is to wait six weeks after giving birth, but if your partner experienced any trauma or tearing, it could be longer. In some cases, much longer. Her body isn't the same, and she may feel self-conscious about that, too. The first time is a little scary even if she's feeling okay, so talk about it first, and be gentle. Vaginal dryness is common, especially if she is breast-feeding, so if you get things going, keep lube at the ready.

# RECOVERY

In China, some new moms practice *zuo yue zi*, or "sitting in," the month after birth. They stay at home and rest while a live-in assistant cooks and handles childcare. South Korea takes this idea of sitting in a step further with *joriwon*, an all-inclusive resort for postnatal care. For two weeks, mothers' bodies are pampered and all meals are provided, along with massages, yoga, laundry, and housekeeping. The Netherlands has a service called Kraamzorg that sends a maternity nurse over every day for up to two weeks after birth. The nurse not only checks in on you and the baby and answers questions, but does household chores and runs to the grocery store. The service is reimbursed almost entirely by basic health insurance policies.[1]

You get the idea—support systems exist because recovery after birth takes time and help. Care in the US is not quite so focused on a mom's well-being, and there is certainly no luxurious spa-like environment waiting to welcome you and your newborn.

While a trip to the pediatrician will happen a few days after you go home, the first appointment to check on you may not be for six weeks. Making contact with your care team in the first three weeks is encouraged,[2] but it is not yet a universal standard of care. A bonus of working with a doula is that they typically do a home visit shortly after birth to check in and help out with recovery, breastfeeding, and general well-being. And there are postpartum doulas who can provide extra help if you do not have family around, are a single mom, or your partner has to go back to work. Other than that, unless you utilize telemedicine, tap into your broader network of providers, or organize someone else to help, you're on your own.

Only 60 percent of women attend their six-week postpartum checkup. Letting it slide makes sense deep in newborn land. You're tired, and it's much easier to put aside your own needs than your baby's. But your health is important, too—as a caretaker, food source, and giver of love and affection. The low attendance rate is why the pediatrician will ask how you are doing and if you have enough help. Pediatricians are often the first line of defense in identifying postpartum depression and problems with parents.

When—not if! (take the baby; your provider will love meeting them!)—you attend your postpartum appointment, discussion topics will range from how you are doing physically and checking your incision if you had a C-section or perineal recovery from a vaginal birth, to pregnancy spacing (how long you plan to wait if you're having another child) and birth control, feeding your baby, medical conditions you are managing, and emotional wellness.

## SCREW GETTING YOUR OLD BODY BACK

Your social media feeds are filled with toned abs and perky boobs on infant-toting women wearing bikinis mere weeks after giving birth. So it must be easy to get that body you miss back, right?

Yeah, no. Mommy tucks, Photoshop, personal trainers, good lighting, and strategic angles all make it look a lot easier than it is. And there's another secret. That old body you had before pregnancy? It's gone. Poof. Sorry. Your body will never be exactly the same again.

Your uterus will shrink from watermelon size back to a closed fist just six weeks after birth, which will flatten out your bump considerably.

The most noticeable contraction happens in the first three days, especially during and after breastfeeding. Your abs will begin to knit back together as your uterus contracts, but it takes eight weeks or longer for them to close the gap entirely. Your pelvic floor can take up to a year to recover, as it was stretched to three times its normal limit during pregnancy and birth. If you're breastfeeding, you will hold on to a bit of extra fat until the baby weans. Your thyroid, aka the controller of your metabolism, can experience changes that make it harder for you to lose weight after pregnancy, too.

Instead of pining for the original version, it's time to celebrate body 2.0. Yes, it's a little more stretched, and if you decide to step on a scale (please don't for a while!), the number you'll see will probably be higher than you'd like. But this new body pulled off GROWING AND BIRTHING A HUMAN BEING. So be proud, and cut yourself and that amazing body some freaking slack.

Body dysmorphia is common during and after pregnancy, and can be serious. It can manifest as fear, feelings of lost control, or in conditions like pregorexia, which is anorexia in pregnant and postpartum women. Having trouble relating to physical changes is normal, but if you are obsessing or unable to let things go, talk to someone.

If you're an active person and worked out during pregnancy, the break you need to take during the postpartum period can be difficult, especially if you are itchy to get back to it or feel pressure to shed baby weight. So what can or should you do physically in the first six weeks? The answer varies based on what happened during birth and how you're healing. In the first week, don't plan to do much except walk. In fact, to avoid any issues like prolapse or diastasis, stick to gentle movements for the first six weeks, and don't lift anything heavy other than the baby (challenging if you already have another child at home!). Going too hard too fast can set back your recovery, so take it slow. Walks with the stroller are invigorating (given it's not Minnesota in January), and a great way to soothe a fussy newborn and give you a break from cabin fever.

## COMPLICATIONS

Hearing that your body and vagina stretch *a lot* during pregnancy and birth is no surprise. But there are three conditions that top the list of dirty, dirty postpartum secrets no one tells you. Perineal and vaginal tearing, diastasis recti, and pelvic organ prolapse affect millions of women to varying degrees, yet awareness of these conditions is very low.

France's *la rééducation périnéale*, aka pelvic floor rehabilitation program, is a standard of care for all women who give birth. Though there is no similar support in the US, consider channeling your inner French girl and make an appointment with a pelvic floor therapist. Unless they are out of network or don't accept it, insurance should cover these appointments. It's also important to get back into your Kegels and pelvic floor strengthening as soon as you can after giving birth. Even though you probably won't be able to feel them working for a while, trust that they are!

### *Dealing with diastasis*

No matter how diligent you are, that stubborn post-pregnancy pooch can hang around for months and sometimes years after birth. Diastasis recti happens when the tissue in your abdominal muscles weakens and stretches during pregnancy to accommodate your growing baby. More than 60 percent of pregnant women experience diastasis in some degree, and it's not completely preventable.

The effects are not just cosmetic. A diastasis diagnosis can mean worse posture, lower-back pain, pelvic prolapse, increased risk of hernia, and more frequent instances of incontinence. Ugh. Your provider may check for it at your six-week appointment by measuring the width between your lower abs with their fingers. A one- or two-finger-width split is normal, and will heal on its own. If it's wider, you may need to do some work to bring your abs back together.

The most successful way to treat diastasis is not to work hard at the gym; it's to target and strengthen your transverse abdominis (TVA).[3] Think of the TVA as your body's corset. It is the deep abdominal muscle that wraps around your torso. You'll learn more about this muscle if you work with a pelvic floor PT, and postpartum Pilates is another excellent way to learn more about this work. If you're ready to fire up your TVA, one favorite move is below.

## Spinal Compressions

- Lie on your back with knees bent and feet hip-distance apart.
- Press your spine into the floor as if you're smashing a bug with your lower back.
- Hold this abdominal contraction for three to four breaths, breathing in your upper ribs.
- Relax and release your abs.
- Repeat eight to ten times.

Just as important as rehabbing your TVA and pelvic floor is avoiding movements that make the splitting worse. Traditional ab exercises (sit-ups, crunches, roll-ups, curls), backbends, spinal extensions, and planks are some of the worst offenders. Avoid heavy lifting for the first six to eight weeks, and try to avoid straining, which means eating a fiber-rich diet to prevent constipation.

Postpartum belly binding and wrapping is a tradition in many cultures around the world. And there is proof that during C-section recovery, it can improve walking, control pain, and help overall with patient satisfaction.[4] Let's be clear: This isn't a corset designed to give you a Victorian waist. We are talking about a medical-grade, elasticized, nothing-sexy-about-it binder designed specifically for the postpartum period. You may even be offered one at the hospital. There is some research that shows it can help your abs zip back together. But what you'll hear anecdotally is that binders make you feel more solid and held in while your organs are still all over the place.

*I did not experience any diastasis, which I attribute in part to my careful avoidance of lifting heavy things and crunching motions. Also luck, genetics, and actually knowing about it beforehand. Eight weeks postpartum, I still did the roly-poly sit-up from bed so I didn't put unwelcome pressure on my abs. I used an abdominal binder after my C-section, starting in the hospital and continuing most days for the first few weeks. While I can't attribute my fast recovery to it directly, I did love the way I felt pulled back together, and my abs did flatten out more quickly than I expected. My rib cage did not get that memo and has yet to retreat to its prepregnancy size even months later.*

### Perineal pain and tearing

Nearly all first-time mothers with vaginal births experience some amount of perineal pain and tearing. Often, it means you will leave the hospital with a few stitches. Depending on the severity, activities like using the restroom, laughing, sneezing, and coughing will be painful for a few weeks, and you will experience some incontinence.

There are four classifications of tearing, and first- and second-degree tears are by far the most common. Around 4 percent of all tears are third- or fourth-degree,[5] so when you read about them, don't panic.

- **First-degree:** minor tears of the vagina's mucosal tissue that don't generally require stitches
- **Second-degree:** vaginal tearing plus some perineal tearing that requires stitches
- **Third-degree:** vaginal tearing plus perineal tearing plus anal sphincter tearing that requires stitches and sometimes surgery
- **Fourth-degree:** tear all the way from vagina and perineum to anus requiring stitches and surgery

Though there are now healing foams and liners, bidets, and squirt bottles for a sore perineum, one classic solution is the padsicle. It is exactly what you'd guess—a menstrual pad that you soak in a brew of different healing agents and put into your mesh underwear for cooling relief.

### Padsicle recipe

**Ingredients:**

>4 tablespoons witch hazel (alcohol-free)
>2 tablespoons aloe vera gel
>1 to 2 drops of lavender essential oil
>your favorite menstrual pads
>spray bottle
>freezer bags
>freezer

Mix the witch hazel, aloe, and lavender oil and pour into a spray bottle. Pull out your favorite menstrual pad and spray on a layer of this concoction until it's wet but not soaked. Put the pad in a freezer bag and place it in the freezer. When it chills, ice down your perineum.

If you're not into frozen pads, the best ways to support recovery are to keep things clean and not mess with your stitches, squirt warm water while and after going to the bathroom (bidets are great for this if you want to upgrade your toilet), avoid constipation, sit on a donut pillow, and use a warm compress or sitz bath.

## Pelvic organ prolapse

Women often describe pelvic organ prolapse (POP, the worst possible acronym for this condition) as their vagina falling out or like sitting on a ball. Think of it as a hernia in the vagina. It happens when the bladder, uterus, small intestine, or rectum pushes against the vaginal wall, causing the vaginal wall to bulge outside of the vagina. It occurs most commonly after vaginal childbirth when the pelvic floor ligaments and fascia are stretched and can no longer hold the wall of the vagina up. POP can cause major issues like difficulty urinating and persistent back pain, and impacts the ability to exercise, especially running and jumping. Many sufferers avoid sex or intimacy due to the threat of incontinence.

POP is not a new condition. It is referenced in the Bible and Egyptian hieroglyphics, with proposed treatments ranging from scaring things back into place with a hot poker, to tying a woman to a ladder upside down and shaking it. Thankfully, fumigating your vagina with herbs or dangling from a rope has been replaced by (you guessed it) pelvic floor rehab and surgery. More than two hundred thousand surgeries are performed each year to treat prolapse, and the number is climbing, so much so that there is a new medical subspecialty called female pelvic medicine and reconstructive surgery (FPMRS) within urogynecology.

More than one in five women (that we know about—it's often not reported) experience POP,[6] and the older you are, the more likely it is to happen. It is especially common when women hit menopause due to the drop in estrogen. It is difficult to diagnose because it may not be obvious in exams, or even a part of routine postpartum checkups. If you feel a lot of discomfort, or experience continued incontinence or a backache that won't go away, you should talk to your provider. They'll prescribe PT or a pessary, which is a device inserted into the vagina to support the pelvic organs, before surgery is considered. If you're planning to have more children, many physicians will wait to perform surgery until you are all finished with pregnancy.

## MANAGING YOUR MENTAL HEALTH

Right after birth, estrogen and progesterone drop, and oxytocin surges. This can lead to anxiety and what's known as the "baby blues." The blues don't last forever, but can cause a rough ten or so days of tears, irritability, anxiety, and fatigue. Then they fade away.

Postpartum depression (PPD) is a different story. One in five mothers experiences mild to serious feelings of depression during pregnancy and in the first year postpartum. While shocking enough, this number is assumed to be wildly underreported. Women are more susceptible to depression during times of transition, especially during their reproductive years. There is new evidence that brain chemistry changes in pregnancy and postpartum are significant, and that neurotransmitters, the signals that manage emotion and mental processing, are in states of flux. This means that the mental health changes are physiological, and not due to inadequate or a lack of coping skills.

During the reproductive years, many women see only one practitioner: an ob-gyn. Historically, peripartum mental health has not been a major part of the obstetric curriculum, which means it can often go undetected.[7] However, in California, screening once during pregnancy and postpartum is now a requirement by law that will, hopefully, inspire the rest of the country to make it a standard of care.

The epidemic levels of PPD did not go unnoticed. A task force was assembled to review the most common interventions[8] and better identify those at highest risk. Many methods of dealing with postpartum depression were examined—physical activity, yoga, writing, supplements, and antidepressants. But the most effective method by far was counseling. Women who received one or two forms of counseling were 39 percent less likely to develop PPD.

How do you know if it's a case of the baby blues, or PPD? The first is timing. The baby blues usually stop around two weeks post-birth. PPD can go on for months. Lack of interest in your baby or difficulty bonding, avoiding family and friends, or an inability to take care of yourself or your baby are symptoms to watch for. And if you have suicidal thoughts, cannot stop crying, or consider harming your baby, it's time to get help. Mental health professionals are available in person, via video chat, text, apps, or phone. So are friends and family. Reach out to whichever makes you feel comfortable—but, please, do not try to deal with it by yourself.

## EATING WHILE PARENTING

Gone is the need to avoid sushi and deli meat. So now that you're not pregnant, what should you eat? To the surprise of no one, postpartum dietary recommendations are just as varied as those proposed during pregnancy. Warm cooked foods, bone broth, and plenty of protein and iron-rich items are common to most nutritional plans. The easiest thing to do: If you developed a good routine while pregnant, just continue to eat that way, by mixing lean proteins with whole grains, fresh fruits and vegetables, and dairy.

Even if you feel pressure to lose the baby weight, immediately after birth is not the time to diet or restrict calories, especially if you are breastfeeding. Breastfeeders actually have more nutritional and caloric requirements than pregnant women. What you eat goes into breast milk, and can shape your child's dietary preferences later. Staying well hydrated is key to helping your body heal and produce breast milk, so drink plenty of water throughout the day, too.

If family and friends offer to pitch in, give them your general dietary guidelines and dishes you like but try not to be too picky. If you're not on the meal train, food delivery services and cooking in batches designed to last for several days ensure you always have things around. Speaking of convenience, healthy snacks are another must in this period, so identify a few items that speak to you and buy them in bulk.

Finally, a note on supplements and vitamins. Many women are prescribed an iron supplement to offset deficiencies caused by bleeding during birth. Before you stay on it long-term, have your levels checked to make sure it's actually needed. Iron can cause constipation, and really that's the last thing you want on top of everything else going on down there. Eating iron-rich foods is a better way to build back iron stores anyway. A multivitamin and mineral complex can be beneficial, and if you are breastfeeding, it's recommended to continue the prenatal vitamins until you stop.

## THE RETURN OF YOUR PERIOD, AND WHAT TO DO ABOUT BIRTH CONTROL

Sex may be the last thing on your mind right now. But when you do feel ready to give it a try, think about that friend, family member, or celebrity with kids whose birthdays are close together. Like, *really* close, maybe just a single year apart. Though it sounds crazy, you can get pregnant again as soon as ten days after giving birth.

Breastfeeding is marketed as birth control, and it's true—if you have not had your period since birth and are exclusively breastfeeding, your body likely will not ovulate. But there are strict rules that you have to follow *perfectly* for it to work. Not doing things perfectly is how two in one hundred women get pregnant anyway while exclusively breastfeeding in the first six months.

Breastfeeding is highly effective birth control only if your baby is receiving no other food, formula, or bottles, and you are nursing at least every four hours during the day and every six hours at night. There is no pumping allowed. Also important: It works only during the first six months of a baby's life, or until their diet includes real foods. When executed flawlessly, breastfeeding is as effective as the pill. When it's not, you'll welcome another baby sooner than you planned.

There are plenty of breastfeeding-approved backup birth control choices. Condoms, diaphragms, and cervical caps are all possibilities if you'd rather stay free of extra hormones. The shot, IUDs, implants, and a pill formulation called the minipill are safe-while-breastfeeding hormone-delivery options.

## VISITING HOURS

One nice bonus of having a newborn is that everyone comes to see you, especially in those early weeks, and many times armed with food and presents. Unfortunately, well-meaning, excited friends and family often overstay without considering the stress of hosting while adjusting to life as a new parent. This trend can start in the delivery room and extend long after birth.

You and the baby can get partied out quickly, so before you welcome a parade of people, set expectations. Here are a few things to think about:

- Pediatricians will tell you not to let your guests play hot potato and pass the newborn around, especially if they have germ magnets, aka toddlers, at home. Be prepared for disappointed faces if you tell someone no.
- If you plan to let someone hold the baby, keep hand sanitizer around or direct your guest to wash their hands before picking them up. Newborn pertussis can be fatal, so make sure anyone holding your newborn has had a Tdap vaccine, too.
- The way your parents or in-laws did things may not be the same way you choose to do things. Seeing them holding or feeding your baby differently can be hard to watch. It's even harder not to correct them. Most of the time, it's better to just let them enjoy their time together, unless they are doing something potentially dangerous (like putting a newborn on their stomach to sleep). If they want to learn or are generally open to feedback, have at it.
- The opposite can also happen when your guests provide unwelcome commentary about your parenting style. Rather than silently resenting the

advice giver, if you are on the receiving end of well-intentioned feedback, smile, say thanks, and try to let it go.

- Keep visits short. For friends, an ideal visit duration is around thirty minutes. Family and people who are there to lend a hand can stay longer.
- If you don't want pictures of your baby (or you) posted on social media, let people know.

# YOUR NEW ROOMMATE

**W**e'll get back to you shortly. But since it's a major part of your new existence, you probably have questions about that adorable baby you are getting to know. Speaking of adorable, ever wonder why babies are so cute? Answer: Cuteness is critical to their survival.

Human babies are completely helpless at birth. And just like not knowing what triggers labor, we don't really understand why they are born at such a mental deficit. To give a sense of how underdeveloped a newborn human's brain is compared to other primates, in order to match the cognitive development of a newborn chimpanzee, human gestation would need to be between eighteen and twenty-one months.[1]

The classically held belief around the nine-month timeline is known as the obstetrical dilemma hypothesis. It theorizes that the size of a newborn's brain is 30 percent of an adult's because it has to fit through a narrow pelvis on a body designed to walk upright. Another theory is that the parasite-like relationship between baby and mother is threatened around nine months, when the mother can no longer meet the baby's metabolic needs.

Whatever the reason, it means that functioning as a human is a learned skill, and newborns are unable to communicate their needs in a language more nuanced than whining and howling. To decipher these cries for help, it's useful to understand what their post-uterus world is like.

For a while, a newborn is nostalgic for their old cozy home in your belly, and needs help feeling secure and protected. After nine months of going everywhere with you, motion makes them feel soothed, which means a lot of rocking, walking, swinging, and jiggling. Their behavior beyond crying and sleeping includes burps, hiccups, curling into the fetal position, snuffles, and pauses between breaths for uncomfortable periods of time.

The involuntary, spastic shooting out of arms and legs has a name: the Moro or startle reflex. It is believed to be a primitive survival instinct that alerts the newborn to a loss of balance, which keeps them from losing grip on their mother. It happens randomly and is triggered by a change from one surface to another, unexpected loud noises and changes in light, and anything else that shifts the amount of support they feel. The Moro reflex persists until babies are three to four months and causes fits of crying and can get in the way of sleep. Swaddling is one of the most effective ways to counteract it, as it provides consistent physical support.

Unless you're really good at origami, swaddling perplexes most first-time parents, especially when learning on a squirmy newborn. It may take several tries to find a technique that works, depending on how much your baby enjoys jail-breaking. There are different folding methods of varying complexity, and many, many models and materials on the market, including sleep sack swaddles that require little more than putting it on your baby like pj's and wrapping the Velcro. If you do want to try the traditional muslin or cotton blanket folding method, here is the classic how-to.

## THE CLASSIC DIAMOND SWADDLE TECHNIQUE

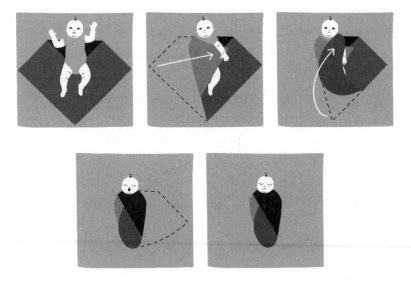

If your baby resists, swaddling may not be for them, as it's meant to provide comfort, not be a punishment. Swaddles should not be used in overly hot climates, or on babies who co-sleep, have a higher risk of SIDS, or have hip issues. As soon as your baby starts rolling over, which can happen as early as eight weeks, it's time to take them out of the swaddle. At that point, there may be a sleep regression due to the wildly flapping arms, so consider transitioning slowly, by reducing usage and leaving one arm out during the daytime so they can get used to it.

Preference for a tight, womb-like environment aside, what about a baby's senses—hearing, seeing, and tasting?

Newborns know their mother's voice straightaway, as they've heard it over and over during pregnancy. They emerge with decent auditory skills, though the fluid in their middle ear makes them most responsive to high-pitched voices—hence their love of baby talk. Other favorite newborn sounds mimic the *shhhhh*s and gurgles of the womb, which is why white noise and shushing are such popular ways to put babies at ease (or to sleep!).

Their visual abilities are not so good for a few months. Newborns can see only up to two feet for the first weeks, and everything looks like a black-and-white movie. Bright lights can cause screaming, so it's wise to keep them out of direct sun. The occasionally cross-eyed gazes deep into your eyes happen because babies LOVE faces. Their second-favorite visuals are high-contrast monochrome patterns and pictures, as they can't detect the nuances of color until around four months.

There's nothing on the menu but breast milk or formula for a while, but babies still come loaded with taste preferences. Sweet always trumps bitter, and newborns turn away from smells and tastes they don't like. What you ate while pregnant and eat now if you're breastfeeding can influence their eventual flavor and food preferences later. So if you want your kid to have an adventurous palate, start now by embracing a diverse (but not gas-causing) diet.

Newborns have a hard time regulating body temperature, so dress them in one more layer than you would wear so they are cozy and warm. Initially, most babies HATE being naked, and will scream when undressed or bathed and during diaper changes. While it's natural to try hacks like wipe warmers to get through this loud and painful period, long-term it's easier to power through until they learn to adjust.

The weird umbilical cord stump will dry up and eventually fall off up to a month after birth. In the meantime, keep the area clean and fold your baby's diaper down so it stays dry and heals. Tummy time should also wait until after the cord drops off.

Now that we know how they see the world, let's learn more about their primary activities. No matter how unique your baby grows to become, infants are limited to sleeping, crying, eating, and soiling diapers for those first months.

*One of Mr. Baby's many nicknames was "little wizard" or "little mage," as his flapping arms looked like he was casting spells on all who passed. Swaddling worked really well for him, though it took five different attempts to find one that he couldn't break out of. When he hit eight weeks, he started rolling, so swaddling had to go. And with it went his formerly long spans of sleep at night, as his flailing limbs woke him up.*

## SLEEPING

Newborns spend eight to ten hours during the day sleeping, and six to eight hours at night (though not consecutively for a while), waking mostly to be fed, burped, and put back down for a nap. They do not emerge from the womb understanding the difference between day and night. In fact, most newborns get the two confused at first, which you may have noted at 3 a.m. if yours is ready to party. One sleeping pro tip is to make the room where they are napping dark even during the daytime so they associate dark with sleep. If it's time to play, make sure it's in a light place. And though it's tempting to talk to them at all times, if a nap or bedtime is happening soon, better to stay quiet and let them relax.

Babies who are ready for sleep may tip you off with a yawn, or by rubbing their eyes, looking away from you, or fussing. It can be irresistible to breastfeed or rock a baby all the way to sleep. However, babies who rely exclusively on a parent or boob to go down may have a hard time going back to sleep if they wake up. It's why most pediatricians recommend letting a baby get sleepy and calm in your arms, but putting them into bed still awake. A bedtime routine can also be beneficial, as it teaches your baby what to expect. At first it probably won't be much — changing a diaper, feeding, and putting them down to sleep. Eventually it can grow to include reading a book or playing soft, calm music as they settle down at night. A white-noise machine can be very helpful early on, especially if it has the librarian setting ("shhh shhh shhh").

There are a lot of rules when it comes to where and how newborns sleep, and many practices are still hotly debated by different groups. In 1992, the American Academy of Pediatrics (AAP) made the "back-to-sleep" recommendation, which advocates that babies sleep on their backs exclusively. It advises against soft surfaces, loose bedding, stuffed toys, blankets, and crib bumpers. Since its publication, the rate of SIDS has dropped more than 50 percent. SIDS rates can also be lower among babies who use pacifiers, though the AAP cautions against using them during the first month or before breastfeeding is established.

While co-sleeping is more convenient, and many parents do it, the AAP advises against it for many of the same reasons relating to SIDS. The crib or bassinet should be in the same room, preferably near your bed, for the first six months. But as nice as baby snuggles can be, all actual sleep is advised to happen separately. This also means that if you have multiples, each baby gets their own sleeping quarters.

Sleeping through the night is generally not a thing until around three months or a baby hits twelve to thirteen pounds. This can vary somewhat based on the baby and what they are fed. Ironically, cutting nap time during the day does not help sleep duration at night. Babies who do not get enough rest during the day can become overtired, and have a harder time staying asleep.

## CRYING

Babies cry for a few reasons: They're hungry, there is a poopy diaper, they are overstimulated, or they hate you. Just kidding! Even if they scream in your face constantly, your baby does not hate you. Crying is their only real way of communicating. Given a little time, you'll understand the difference between whines and *I'm mad* and *something is seriously wrong*. Promise.

Let's pause for a moment on overstimulation, since it can be the trickiest to learn. Overstimulation, or letting your baby go into sensory overload from bright light, too much handling, or staring at something for too long, can stand in the way of developing good sleep habits, and lead to loud, tearful screams. When babies wake up from a sleep cycle, they enter into what is known as a quiet alert phase. During this time they can stare at objects and take in what's happening around them. Next is active alert, when they are moving and responding to sounds and visuals. Then, the worst phase—when they cry.

Some babies also have what's called a "witching hour," or a specific time of day when they seem to cry for no reason. It's most common toward the end of the day, when body temperature is at its peak and your baby is tired, making it tough to relax. Babies make very little melatonin in the first three months of life when this inexplicable crying peaks; this also contributes, since melatonin is responsible for regulating our sleep/wake cycles.

How do you stop a baby from crying? First, identify the problem. If a baby is hungry, crying is actually a late sign, and they might refuse the boob or bottle. Crying during a feeding? Try burping. Pumping legs accompanied by screaming usually means gas, which can be relieved by bicycling their legs. A reliable way to calm a baby down is to go for a walk, as the fresh air can help them relax. Appealing to their love of sucking is another, hence the popularity of pacifiers.

And then there's colic. It's a condition with no known cause (or at least not one that adults understand) that causes crying for hours and hours at a time. You can identify colic using the rule of three: more than three hours of crying per day for more than three days per week for at least three weeks. It usually peaks around six to eight weeks and improves as babies hit three or four months.

If you reach a breaking point during a never-ending spell of crying, take a breather. Ask your partner to take over, or just put the baby down in a safe place like a crib until you can get it together. It's normal to have these moments; just remember, it won't last forever.

*Yes, I googled "Does my baby hate me?" after one particularly epic crying jag. Turns out Mr. Baby did not hate me, he just had really bad gas.*

## SANITATION DUTY

Newborns create an average of five to seven dirty diapers per day. The majority are just wet, but one will likely be poopy. Don't be surprised when you crack open a diaper right after birth and find a disturbing greenish-black, sticky, tar-like substance. It's called meconium, and within a few days, it will transition to a more normal-looking color. Breastfed baby poop has a mustard mush-style texture and can range in hue from classic yellow to seeded dijon. It smells sweet and can be loose and watery. Formula-fed baby poop has a peanut-buttery, solid consistency with a more offensive bouquet and ranges from pale yellow to light brown. Enjoy the lack of foul odor while you can—once they start eating solid foods, it's all downhill in the smell department.

Colors that deviate from this palette may indicate something is wrong. If the poop is green and watery or slimy, it may be a sign of dehydration or a virus. Dry or hard pellets can indicate constipation. And it's time to call the doctor if there is any pink or red. Though it could be blood the infant swallowed from cracked nipples, it can also mean a milk allergy, an infection, or a rectal tear. Same for thick and black after the first few days of meconium, unless you are using iron-fortified formula.

When you're putting on a diaper, be sure it is well sealed and put on straight to avoid as many blowouts as possible. Worried about diaper rash? Make sure your baby's butt is dry and clean after every change. Slathering Aquaphor on your baby's butt and in the creases before you seal it up is another way to keep their skin smooth and diaper rash–free.

Oh, one more unavoidable thing. If you have a boy, more than once, a tiny stream of urine will hit you in the face, or soak your clothes while traversing the ten feet between the changing table and bathtub. There are devices available to help avoid it from getting you straight on (one of which works particularly well), but it's likely to happen at least once.

## FEEDING TIME

In the early weeks, your baby will eat a lot—between eight and twelve times per day. Why so frequently? Your baby's stomach is really, really tiny at birth. On day one, it can hold a little over one teaspoon of milk and is around the size of a marble. By day three, it's around the size of a Ping-Pong ball. And at one month it is the size of an egg. For comparison, your stomach is around the size of a clenched fist and can expand three to four times its size.

Whether you're breastfeeding or bottle-feeding, meeting your newborn's dietary needs is a full-time job. Each feeding, which in those first months is every two to three hours, takes twenty to thirty minutes to finish. And the clock on the next feeding doesn't start when your baby has had enough. It starts when the boob or bottle first entered their mouth, meaning at most you'll have around two and a half hours before you do it all again.

Now let's get to the meat. People probably asked during pregnancy whether you would breastfeed, and why not if you said no. This more than any other early decision related to your baby's care will stimulate the most polarizing opinions and judgment.

Breastfeeding advocates have trumpeted "breast is best" for decades. These groups, many of whom passionately defend a woman's right to choose, are the first to say there is only one right choice when it comes to feeding babies. Today, breastfeeding is tantamount to social proof of "good" parenting, the implicit judgment being that you are a bad parent if you don't. This external pressure forces new mothers to feel they have absolutely no choice but to do it, regardless of their personal circumstances or challenges.

But breastfeeding wasn't always in fashion.

In the 1950s and 1960s, formula was in vogue, and as a result, by 1972, only 22 percent of babies were breastfed.[2] Then, in 1974, the infamous *Baby Killer* report[3] was published. It detailed the shady promotion and sales of formula in developing countries, and triggered a mass boycott of Nestlé products around the world. A few years later, in 1981, there were more than sixty-six thousand infant formula–related deaths in low- and middle-income countries, caused by mixing powdered formula with contaminated water.[4] As a result, by 1982, 61 percent of mothers initiated breastfeeding, and levels have only risen in the years since.

The massive $70 billion global formula market is growing, primarily due to women's increasing participation in the workforce.[5] Almost all the formula in the US is manufactured and sold by just three companies— Abbott, Mead Johnson, and Nestlé. Formula research supporting its nutritional qualities is often funded by these companies, too.

Breastfeeding is free, in dollars and of these sticky issues, right? Well, it's free only if your time isn't worth anything. And though it pales in comparison to formula's market size, selling breastfeeding accessories ain't a shabby business either. Also driven by the rise of female employment, it is projected to reach more than $2.5 billion by 2026.[6] Pump manufacturers fund research into breastfeeding, touting pumping's benefits and that of the vacuum effect on breast milk expression.

There are many reasons to breastfeed, and it's a wonderful way to bond with your baby. Breastfed babies may have a reduced risk of asthma, respiratory infections, SIDS, diabetes, childhood leukemia, eczema, IBD, and even obesity.[7] Just like what you eat when your baby is in utero, the composition of breast milk also influences future food preferences and eating behaviors.[8]

Breastfeeding is also good for moms. After birth, it decreases the amount of postpartum blood loss and helps the uterus return to its prepregnancy state more quickly, and later could lower the risk of ovarian and breast cancers, high blood pressure, and type 2 diabetes.[9]

However, exclusively breastfed babies are twice as likely as formula-fed babies to be readmitted to the hospital in the first month after birth.[10] This is due to dehydration and jaundice, both of which are signs of underfeeding.

The official recommendation from most medical groups is

exclusive breast milk for the first six months of life, and breastfeeding alongside other foods from six months to one year.[11] However, the United States has one of the least friendly parental leave policies of any developed nation, so this is a challenge for many families. Only 13 percent of American workers receive paid family leave,[12] and a quarter of new moms return to work just two weeks after birth. The dearth of leave and family-friendly legislation means it can be difficult for working women to stick to breastfeeding guidelines—even those who desperately want to.

Rarely do companies provide on-site day care or other resources for new mothers to breastfeed their babies at work—they offer pumping policies at best. While pumping allows women to keep up their milk supply and provides for bottle-feedings, it does not allow for bonding time. Even if you decide to pump at work, many workplaces do not comply with rules to allot time and dedicated space (much less a refrigerator for milk storage) during the workday, as enforcement of these regulations is nearly impossible. Ironically, investing in lactation support is good for business: For every $1 spent, there is a $2 to $3 return.[13]

There is another problem with the all-or-nothing breastfeeding narrative. Some women, due to low production or other anatomical or physiological factors, cannot breastfeed enough to sustain their babies. There are also issues like tongue-tie, which can impede a baby's ability to latch. And let's not forget the parents who adopt, have cancer, or use a gestational carrier. Donor milk is an option, but it doesn't work for all families.

Here is the state of the baby-feeding union in the US: 83 percent of babies start out on breast milk, and only 58 percent are still breast-fed partially at six months. The number dips to 36 percent at one year. One in six babies supplements with formula within two days of birth. And the number one reason women stop breastfeeding? The return to work. Issues with milk supply and latching, infant nutrition and weight, concern around medications and their side effects, and lack of support from family contribute, too.

Just as with birth, the best-laid breastfeeding ambitions do not always work perfectly. So if you find yourself disappointed, try to put aside those feelings and do your best. Whether you choose to exclusively breastfeed, use breast milk in combination with formula, or go with formula only, choose what works best for you and your family, and remember fed is best.

### How does breastfeeding actually work?

The actual mechanics of breastfeeding are fascinating. The two hormones that affect breastfeeding are prolactin and oxytocin. Oxytocin, also known as the love hormone, makes the milk flow and fill the ducts. It is also responsible for helping shrink your uterus after birth.[14]

When you start the feed, the baby attaches to the breast and stretches the nipple, while cupping their tongue around the sides beneath the milk ducts. They use suction to press the nipple against their palate, which stimulates the oxytocin reflex and the flow of milk. When the latch is good, the suckling can be pleasurable. You can see and hear the baby swallow, sometimes pausing to allow the ducts to fill again. When the baby is satisfied, they will usually pull off on their own. It's important to let them stay on until they let go, as the end of a breastfeeding session is when the fat-rich hindmilk flows out.

With a good latch, the baby takes in not just the nipple, but also the areola and surrounding tissue, with a wide-open mouth. The chin should be touching or almost touching the breast, and more of the areola should be visible above the baby's top lip than below the lower lip. If only the nipple is in the baby's mouth, they cannot access the ducts to press and express milk. If you have a bad latch, it's best to try again. Break the latch by putting your pinky into your baby's mouth, hooking it over the top of the nipple, and very gently pulling it away.

### Lactation consultant pro tips

Breastfeeding seems like it should all just work, right? You present the boob to the baby, and they latch on correctly every time, then stop when they're done. Unfortunately, the first days of breastfeeding can be tough, which is why many hospitals now employ a team of lactation consultants to get you through the early adjustment period. After you leave the hospital, they are available via telemedicine and for in-home visits. Here are a few things you'll likely hear them say if you work together:

- Set a timeline goal for how long you'd like to breastfeed, but be flexible if things aren't working.
- Pump from the beginning to stimulate supply.
- Don't use a pacifier during the early weeks while trying to establish the latch.
- Drink water.
- Get plenty of rest (sleep when the baby sleeps!).

### *Breastfeeding complications (and what to do about them)*

Lactation struggles and their remedies are covered in the first-known medical encyclopedia, Egypt's Papyrus Ebers, dating to 1500 BCE.[15] Wet nurses were frequently utilized in the case of low supply, or inability to nurse, up until the 1900s.[16] From warming the bones of a swordfish in oil and rubbing the mother's back with it, to giving her fragrant bread to eat while rubbing her breasts with the poppy plant, history is full of creative (and sometimes strange) workarounds for breastfeeding challenges.

Struggles with breastfeeding can happen for a number of reasons. It can be as simple as a bad latch or bad positioning. Insufficient glandular tissue and hypoplasia are known causes of low supply. Hormones and illness can also affect how things go, as can breast surgery (augmentations, lifts, reductions, or reconstructions) since it influences the nerves and ducts required for milk production. The most problematic surgeries are implants above the muscle, and those that involve the areola and nipple, as the nerves in the nipple signal your brain to release oxytocin to get milk flowing. How much milk you are able to produce and release depends on how well the nerves and ducts repaired themselves during your recovery.

Having a baby with tongue-tie—when the tissue anchoring the base of the tongue is too tight—can also hurt supply. It affects how the baby moves their tongue, making it difficult to latch and stimulate the breast properly to encourage milk production. There is a procedure to fix problematic cases called "snipping" (which is exactly what it sounds like), but it is painful and sometimes babies grow out of the issue. Tongue-tie is generally more common in boys than in girls.

Today's options to improve supply go beyond rubbing your body with fish oil or flower petals (but hey, try it if you want!). Since the Internet probably knows about your new addition, ads for mysterious supercharged-milk-supply products, or galactagogues, may be rampant in your feeds. Though it sounds more like a way to take your breasts to space, galactagogues are foods, drugs, and herbs that are supposed to increase breast milk production.

There is no medical evidence that, beyond a placebo effect, galactagogues make a real difference. Trials to date have not been well controlled, or have small sample sizes. Unless you are pumping and then bottle-feeding, it's also impossible to tell how much milk is actually making it to the baby during each session. Lactation consultants recommend trying repositioning, more frequent pumping, breast compression, and skin-to-skin first. In more extreme cases, there are also prescription medications that are proven to boost supply.

Anecdotally, people swear by these mega milk-producing substances. If you're curious and want to give them a shot, fenugreek, alfalfa, blessed thistle, goat's rue, and moringa are the top herbal supplement picks and primary ingredients in mother's milk tea, tinctures, and bars. Chat with your doctor to ensure they don't cause side effects or interactions with other medications you're taking—as with the supplement industry at large, there is no real regulation of galactagogues.

Eating specific foods is another route to increased supply. The most commonly cited milk boosters are almonds, anise, barley, brewer's yeast, chickpeas, coconut, dill, millet, oats, and rice. All of these are nutritious and fine to mix into your daily routine.

Another, less nutritious but popular solution for low production is beer. One of the polysaccharides in the barley used to make beer seems to stimulate prolactin. Drinking a single beer right after a feeding or pumping session is best, as it takes around two hours to clear out of your bloodstream and breast milk. But don't overdo it—alcohol reduces production, so having one is enough.

Just like in so many areas of maternal health, research is just not conclusive as to how many women have low supply and why. So if you've tried everything, are pumping and hand-expressing around the clock, have worked with a lactation consultant, are eating your weight in oatmeal bars, and still nothing is happening, you may want to consider plan B.

Breast maintenance issues and infections can cause speed bumps, too. So take good care of your breasts, and use lanolin or coconut oil to keep your nipples moist and free of cracks.

### Get pumped up

If you can't be with your baby 24/7, you may need to pump your breast milk. We already covered how to select a breast pump model, but here's a refresher. Insurance is required to provide one gratis, so contact them to explore your options and order. There are new hands-free models that make the job easier, but insurance doesn't pay for them and they are generally less powerful. Most pumps require holding the flanges in place or use of a pumping bra, as the seal is not strong enough to avoid leakage on its own. On that note, pumping requires accessories, and the Internet is there for it. Many of them, from bags to coolers to cover-ups, are now stylish and discreet.

The process of pumping is, well, strange. You'll finally understand what it feels like to be a dairy cow, and will get used to the gentle rhythmic *whoosh whoosh whoosh* and the hypnotic look of your nipples expanding and squirting streams of milk from tiny holes you didn't even know existed.

Whether you're out and about, at work, or just at home, here are the top mom-approved pumping tips and tricks:

- Keep an extra set of flanges and pump parts at work, and store them in a plastic bag in the refrigerator or cooler. This way, you only have to clean up once per day and the drips are contained.
- Button-down shirts make things easier for speedy pumping and breastfeeding. Your breastfeeding cover-up works to keep things undercover, too.
- Carry an extra shirt or paper towels to help with unexpected leakage and drips.
- Having trouble with letdown? Look at photos or a video of your baby for help, or consider carrying a onesie that smells like them.
- Slather on the nipple cream to keep things moist before and after pumping. Many are baby-friendly, so you won't have to wash it off if you're still nursing.
- Consider keeping a manual hand pump around. They're cheap and way easier to use on the go.
- Buy backup parts for your pump, and keep them clean, especially the tiny plastic membranes, which can easily go down the drain while washing.
- If you don't have access to a refrigerator to store milk or room to store a mini-model at your desk, tote a cooler with ice packs from home.
- Though you'll have to pay for it, consider buying a second pump that just lives at work, especially if you take public transportation.

So what to do with all of this extra milk? Freeze it, baby. Getting a stash going is great before you go back to work, for the times you won't be with your baby, and in case your supply drops. When you bag it up, label it with the date pumped, and fill in varying amounts so nothing goes to waste—for example, one-ounce and two-ounce bags are useful for top-offs, whereas a four-ounce bag can get you through a whole feeding. Mind the fill lines, since milk expands while freezing. Pumped milk stays good at room temperature for four hours, in a refrigerator for up to three days, in your normal freezer for six months, and in a deep freezer for up to twelve months.

When you are ready to thaw, you can put breast milk in the refrigerator for twelve hours, or hold it under warm running water. Never use the microwave or boiling water, as they can damage breast milk's nutritional properties. And when that liquid gold finally goes into the bottle, think swirled, not shaken, if the fat has separated.

## The f-word

Ingredient-wise, formula contains the same basic vitamins and nutrients as breast milk but lacks the rich antibodies. Most formulas are based on cow's milk or soy milk, which require processing to meet the needs of human infants, and are iron-fortified—an ingredient not found in breast milk.

So how do you pick a good formula? The answer isn't straightforward, as much of what actually makes a formula good for your baby is what works for their specific digestive system.

There is a perception that, like croissants and wine, European formula is better because there is more stringent regulation, and the ingredients are cleaner. That idea is not entirely without merit, for three reasons: (1) all formulations are organic, since the EU dictates that there are no detectable levels of pesticide residue in formula, (2) the cows are all grass-fed and live on biodynamic farms, and (3) corn syrup is not an ingredient. If you do choose a European formula, pay attention to the stage it's meant for, as the nutrition is tailored to that age range, and ensure you have a good label translation (unless your German is better than mine) so you know what you're getting. Because they aren't FDA-approved, your pediatrician may not be amped about a European formula, so be prepared to make your case if it comes up.

Formula comes in three types: powder, concentrated liquid, and ready-to-use. Powder is the easiest for travel, and the cheapest, but can cause constipation and is less easy to digest. You'll need to mix it with water before feeding your baby. Concentrated is more expensive than powder, but still requires that you add water. Ready-to-use is the priciest and least convenient of all, but is best for infants with picky digestive systems. Instead of buying a huge container, ask your pediatrician for recommendations. Try each type for at least three days before rejecting it as an option, as it takes time for your baby's digestive system to adjust.

The other challenge with formula is bottle/baby fit. There are many, many bottle options—low-flow, fast-flow, vented, glass, plastic, silicone, flat or natural nipples . . . the list goes on. As with every other accessory, it comes down to your baby's individual preferences. If you have a gassy or colicky baby, a low-flow or vented bottle is a good choice. For a baby who loves the boob, try a breast-like nipple. Pumping frequently? You can find a container that doubles as a bottle so you can pump, screw on the nipple, and feed.

Though it is still highly regulated and tough to break into, the formula market is finally seeing innovation from startups. From reproducing the functional sugars found naturally in human breast milk to reformulating them from the ground up, the quality and options for formula-fed babies are only getting better.

### Donor milk

"Liquid gold," they call it. And at $3 to $5 per ounce, the name is fitting. There is a whole regulated industry around donor breast milk for people who need a bridge to breastfeeding or just do not want to use formula. It relies on mothers who have extra production and a milk bank to receive, process, and redistribute the milk. Here's how it works.

To donate at a licensed bank, mothers are given a health screening, including a blood test to ensure they don't have any diseases like HIV or hepatitis that can be transferred to the baby. If approved, the donor pumps and freezes her extra supply (most banks will take deep-frozen milk up to six months after it's pumped) and ships it to the bank in a cooler. The bank then puts the donor milk through a process called Holder pasteurization (HoP). During HoP, the breast milk is slowly unfrozen and heated to 62.5 degrees Celsius for half an hour. The milk is then tested for any pathogens, bacteria, or viruses before it is refrozen and distributed to families in need.

HoP is used around the world to make human milk safe for infants, but there is a downside, namely that it reduces the beneficial properties.[17] The pasteurization process lowers the concentration of many vitamins (vitamin C is eliminated entirely), as well as fat. It also reduces lactoferrin, a protein that binds iron, which can fight germs and is thought to stimulate intestinal development. Some studies are starting to show that HoP may even be worse than a commercial preparation, meaning you might be better off just using a high-quality formula.

Insurers will cover the cost of donor milk for preemies, but the majority of parents have to pay out-of-pocket. Considering that a one-month-old baby can drink thirty ounces of breast milk per day, at $3 to $5 per ounce, exclusively using donor milk means your tab will be thousands of dollars per month.

Inevitably, the high cost of licensed-donor milk means there is a gray market online and a local cottage industry of mothers who sell or donate directly. Though it's not technically illegal, if you are considering this even with close friends or family, you should know the risks. There is no guarantee that what you'll receive ordering online is even human milk.[18] You won't know with certainty the donor's health history or lifestyle, if she's been exposed to any harmful bacteria or other substances, or what, if any, medications will be passed to your baby. Even with the most well-intentioned donors, this contamination can happen accidentally from poor storage or sterilization methods.

The Human Milk Banking Association of North America is the largest network of licensed milk banks, if you'd like to explore your options.

*Our breastfeeding journey was also (surprise, surprise) not perfect.*

*After a C-section, it can take a few extra days for milk to come in. Not an uncommon occurrence, after the flood of medications during surgery, pressure put on breast tissue by water retention, and the general lack of rest and sleep. I lost quite a bit of blood after mine, and was pretty anemic on top of everything else. Mr. Baby also had tongue-tie, which meant it could have been challenging for him to latch. Lucky for us, that didn't stop him, perhaps in part because, according to the nurses and LCs, I had "perfect breastfeeding nipples." Definitely one of the oddest compliments I've ever received.*

*Mr. Baby's patience ran out after two days of nothing. I worked with a lactation consultant and started a regimen known as the triple feed to stimulate the flow of milk. This involved feeding the baby, then hand-expressing, then pumping, every two to three hours. Try as I might, even with a hospital-grade pump, I could coax nothing more than a few beads of colostrum out, which I gathered and fed to him with a plastic spoon.*

*All babies lose weight after birth, but once it exceeds 10 percent, I knew from my research that the hospital would encourage temporary formula supplementation. When the pediatrician told us Mr. Baby's weight was now down 12 percent, we agreed to try it. After that first formula feeding with a plastic syringe, the screaming stopped, and he finally slept longer than fifteen minutes at a time. I still did all the milk-stimulating things, but with that little boost his weight stabilized, and we got to go home.*

*Conversations with friends prepared me for the reality that breastfeeding is a full-time job. Stories of mastitis and pumping in closets and leaking breasts and bleeding nipples frankly had me dreading it. On the first point, they were right. I spent a solid eight to ten hours every day in various states of feeding and pumping. But I loved breastfeeding. The time with Mr. Baby was magical. He made adorable happy feeding noises, he snuggled into my chest, and I got high on baby head every time we hung out. Pumping, on the other hand, was not my favorite. It was messy and inconvenient and made me feel like a bovine slave.*

*Around five weeks, we hit another snag. Mr. Baby's gas was so bad that he couldn't sleep. He screamed and pistoned his legs in and out, and no amount of burping, rocking, or gas-reducing drops did a thing about it. I changed my diet and ate the blandest foods possible. When that didn't help, I suspected that, like me, he had a sensitive stomach and possibly colic. We found an easy-to-digest formula, and within a day of substitution, he started sleeping again. I continued to pump, and filled the freezer with milk that he could enjoy once his stomach matured. After the gas subsided, we slowly added breast milk to his formula and started breastfeeding again until we found the right balance.*

*Even with pumping, from the beginning, my supply couldn't keep up with his hunger level, and it continues to be unimpressive. When I spoke to my panel of experts, they suggested that could be due in part to the much higher than normal blood loss I experienced during birth, which led to low iron levels and extra medications. Supplementation gets a bad rap, especially as it relates to supply, but in our case, it was necessary.*

*Since I'm writing in real time and my deadline is twelve weeks postpartum, I can't tell you how or when my breastfeeding journey ends. Only that I'm still giving it my best shot.*

## PERCENTILES AND MILESTONES

Figuring out sleeping, eating, crying, and bowel movements will keep you plenty busy in the first months. But the next thing that is probably occupying your mind (beyond how to handle the never-ending sleep deprivation) is how your baby is growing and developing.

Ultrasounds during pregnancy were the first time you encountered percentiles for height, weight, and head circumference. And now that your baby is out of the womb, you'll encounter them again at well-baby appointments. The pediatrician will take these measurements and plot them on a chart. Where they fall on that chart compared to other babies of the same age dictates the percentile. If your baby's weight falls in the sixtieth percentile, it means 40 percent of babies at that age weigh more and 60 percent weigh less. Though being too far on either end of the spectrum can be problematic, what actually matters is that your baby's growth follows a curve and continues at a steady, predictable rate over time.

Developmental milestones are another way of evaluating how your baby is progressing. Less than half of pediatricians use them in appointments, as they are not a foolproof way of identifying issues or even fairly judging development. In fact, the four most commonly used developmental checklists are pretty inconsistent.[19] While each list features at least 170 milestones, only 40 are common to all four lists, and barely half of those have the same target age for each milestone. For example, one list expects a child's ability to dress and undress to happen at thirty-six months. On another, it's not until month sixty.

Not mapping exactly to these milestones causes a lot of anxiety for parents. And it shouldn't. They are meant to be long-term goals and averages, so try to focus on the big picture.

## A QUICK NOTE ON PARENTING STYLES

Baby cages suspended from the sides of buildings were thought to be an acceptable way to ensure babies got enough fresh air in the 1930s. And there is almost certainly something your parents or grandparents did that you would not dream of doing with your child. So it's safe to say that parenting trends come and go. How you choose to raise your baby is a decision only you and your partner can make. But since it's no doubt on your mind, here is a quick overview of two parenting frameworks in the zeitgeist.

In the US, the most commonly referenced categorizations are known as Baumrind's Parenting Styles. Coined by Diane Baumrind, a developmental psychologist, in the 1960s, they are organized based on variance in communication, nurturance, expectations, and discipline styles. Authoritarians are high on expectations and low on flexibility, and use punishment to enforce desired behavior. Permissive parents let their kids do what they want, are warm and nurturing, and often act more like friends than parents. Uninvolved parents are just that—they give a lot of latitude to their kids and stay out of the way, sometimes due to lack of interest, or because they are just unsure of what to do. Authoritative parents are direct about expectations, clear communicators, nurturing, and include their children in goal- and decision-making. Most research shows that authoritative parenting is the most beneficial style.

The siren song of European child-rearing methods promising perfectly behaved kids in restaurants also may have piqued your interest. As the most commonly referenced of these models, let's take a peek at the stereotypical guidelines of French parenting:

- **No means no.** Be consistent in your discipline and let your child know who is in charge.
- **Self-play and independence.** Your child should be able to entertain him- or herself at times, and not lose it every time your attention is elsewhere.

- **Make time for adults.** Spending time with others who are not your child means a more balanced family where your child doesn't think they are the center of the universe.
- **Teach patience and keep a schedule.** No interruptions, stay on a consistent eating schedule, and wait your turn.
- **Eat what the family eats.** No special food.
- **No baby talk.** Talk to your kids with the same tone of voice you would your partner, and in the same language.

Whether you disagree with the French, or don't identify exactly with any of Baumrind's categorizations, as with pregnancy, and birth, and everything else that happens in this process, what's most important is finding a parenting style that feels right for your family. If you do it all again, you'll find that what works for a first child often doesn't for the second. The two babies will be different, and you will be going through it as a seasoned parent.

# TRANSITIONS

L ike birth, becoming a parent doesn't always line up with the image you had in your head. Maybe you secretly wanted a girl but got a boy. Perhaps you fantasized about bonding during breastfeeding, but that same son won't latch and you have to pump and bottle-feed. Your dreams of being surrounded by friendly moms may be dashed by someone's judgment about your need to bottle-feed. And when you share with your partner, perhaps they don't say the perfect thing to make you feel better.

Once you get the all-clear from your doctor to resume physical activity, your wavering confidence might get in the way of enjoying the things you used to do. Whether that's yoga or having sex, your relationship with your body is different. Balancing your baby, your partner, work, and yourself (never mind a social life) has to happen in the tiny windows between feedings and naps. And it can be really hard to express any ambivalence you may be feeling about your new role as a parent to friends and colleagues—it's *supposed* to be a happy time, right? After all, you have a new baby! You're a MOM. Isn't it all delightful and great?

Yes. And no.

The transition to motherhood involves obvious physical and

lifestyle changes, but there is a lot going on in that mind of yours, too. We know that it takes around two years after birth for your brain to go back to its prepregnancy size. But that's not where the gray matter changes end. The stereotypical mothering behaviors like fierce protectiveness, worry, and love for your baby have neurological roots. And that hamster wheel in your head telling you over and over to make sure the baby is breathing while they sleep or that worries about leaving them at home with someone who isn't you is hard to stop sometimes.

This identity shift is known as matrescence, and it is yet another uncharted and poorly researched part of this process. The amygdala is an almond-shaped set of neurons deep in the brain's medial temporal lobe that drives emotional reactions and processes memory. Amygdala activity is higher in the months after childbirth, and drives mothering behaviors by making you more sensitive to your baby's needs. One study[1] recorded strong brain response in mothers when looking at their own smiling babies versus those who were unfamiliar. That positive ping was also tied to lower anxiety and symptoms of depression, and, scientifically, most resembles falling in love. Which, in a way, it is.

This love you feel, which will only grow, is hard to put aside when it comes time to return to an office.

## GOING BACK TO WORK

Break out the waterproof mascara. For many new mothers, and their partners, the transition back to full-time work feels almost as hard as recovering from birth. If you had the opportunity to spend weeks or months with your baby after birth as the primary caregiver, the idea of leaving them with someone else or in day care can be heartbreaking. Especially since they are only getting more interesting and aware of the world just as you have to do it.

To help with this inevitably difficult period, here are a few of the top pro tips from career coaches.

### Prepare to go back before you actually go back.

Maybe you've been keeping an eye on your inbox throughout your maternity leave. Maybe not. Rather than returning to hundreds or thousands of messages the day you go back to the office, try to get a jump on it and at least scan for what's most important ahead of time. You can also schedule a quick catch-up with your team or boss before your planned return to see what's changed while you were out.

### Plan your first day back in the middle of the week.

Rather than diving right into a full workweek, start on a Wednesday, or even Thursday. The staggered week provides a soft start so you aren't away from your baby five full days in a row.

### Ease into it.

Keep your schedule as open and flexible as possible. While going back part-time might seem appealing, it means you'll miss meetings and may make it harder to reintegrate with the team.

### Talk to your manager and team.

This is another do-it-before-you-actually-go-back task that can set the stage for a successful return. Be realistic about your life, your responsibilities, and what you can and cannot do. Make your work hours and parenting responsibilities clear, and acknowledge how you will cope with emergencies as they come up. If you plan to work from home more (if that's an option), now is a great time to carve out that schedule. This maneuver will help you feel better about what you're committing to do, but will also help your manager and colleagues to calibrate their expectations (and requests) properly.

### Preview (and plan) your work wardrobe.

Even a few months postpartum, you won't look exactly as you did before you were pregnant, and your clothes will not fit the same way.

The last thing you'll want to do in the morning when you head back to the office is stress about what to wear, so do a wardrobe audit a few weeks beforehand so you can pull together and plan a few outfits. This is especially useful on the mornings after your baby hasn't slept, and you don't have time to think about it.

### Ask for help.

More than ever, employers want (and are incentivized) to bring back working moms. This means there are an increasing number of workplaces that provide transitional support to make sure you feel confident in your return, and can focus on your job rather than worrying about your childcare. As long as it doesn't become the new normal, asking for a little flexibility and assistance and understanding in those early days is fine.

### Be open with your partner.

While it may seem most critical that you squeeze in every available moment with your baby before and after work, don't forget about your partner. The transition back to work is a big one for them, too, and involves more responsibility. Keep the lines of communication open, and if you need help—ask. Don't forget to see how they are doing, too. If you're a calendar junkie, throw a meeting on your shared calendar to check in, or try to make it out for a date night when you can.

### Introduce a bottle early.

Even if you are exclusively breastfeeding, at some point you will have to pump to keep up supply or let someone else feed the baby during an afternoon or evening out. Getting your baby used to a bottle before you actually have to go back to work helps make this transition less difficult. Not to mention that it allows your partner the opportunity to try out feeding, which is a great way for them to bond.

### *Practice your morning and evening routines.*

If going back to work is going to meaningfully change your schedule, try a few dry runs with your partner. This will reduce stress and prevent some shock to your system. It will also help you foresee any scheduling difficulties or hiccups with your proposed plan.

### *Stick to a schedule.*

If there are certain evenings each week that you know you or your partner will need to work late, set a calendar that allows both of you to have that flexibility without resenting the other. Shared calendars that list childcare information and any other events are one lightweight way to keep track. There are also plenty of apps that allow this type of collaboration.

## MOM GUILT

Going back to work, or doing anything that doesn't involve your baby, comes with another mental hurdle: mom guilt. Everyone feels shades and different degrees of it, and it doesn't go away when your baby grows into a toddler or goes to school.

Your baby will change. A lot. Every single day in those early months. They're learning to be a human, after all, which it turns out is a long, drawn-out process. Your baby's face, mannerisms, behaviors, sounds, and everything else will change as they grow out of the newborn phase into a more sentient human. It's hard to imagine missing a moment of it. But unless you plan to never leave your child's side, you will miss something eventually.

Another hard thing: If you utilize childcare, whether it's a nanny or day care, your baby will have other close relationships. There may even be moments when it seems like they prefer that person to you. *Cringe.* But as with pregnancy, raising a child is a marathon, not a sprint. You are stuck with each other for the rest of your lives. The caregiver? Not so much.

It's natural to feel jealous or sad or some combination of a hundred conflicting emotions simultaneously. Already in it? You may already be familiar with several of the following runaway thought trains. Not there yet? Read and prepare.

### I'm going to miss everything!

The idea that you wouldn't witness your baby's first steps because you're at work is enough to reduce many parents to tears. And while that could happen, it's just as likely you'd miss it being in a different room or during a run to the grocery store. There are so many developmental milestones during your baby's life that you cannot possibly catch them all.

### My baby is different with me now that I'm back at work.

Your baby will be different as they grow through stages no matter what you do. And letting your baby get to know new people is good for their development. Some babies are timid and shy; others will instantly go to a new person. If your baby is the former, gradual introduction to new adults and other infants is a better way to socialize. But in general, after the first few weeks, exposing them to different people and caretakers helps with long-term growth.

### I can't imagine sending my baby to day care, or letting someone else take care of them.

This is another tough one if you've had the opportunity to spend months at home as the primary caregiver. Hopefully, before you gave birth you had time to carefully vet the person or place who will be responsible for your baby. To help with the transition, and to ease your own fears, you may want to take your baby to day care yourself or have the nanny over once or twice before you have to leave your baby solely in their care. You'll be able to see how the caregiver actually works, ask any remaining questions, and witness how your baby does in their new environment.

### After all that hard work, my milk supply is going to completely dry up.

While it's true that workplaces don't support real bring-your-baby-to-work breastfeeding, they do have to legally provide time and space for pumping, which, done regularly, should ensure consistent supply. You can pump right after breastfeeding (an old trick to make your body think you need to make more milk), before you head to work, and as many times as you need to during the day. You'll also need to stick to your guns with scheduling (this is where those prebooked calendar blocks you put into place come in handy), because skipping or changing the time you pump will impact your supply. If people try to schedule meetings during those blocks, remind them that pumping is your legal right. Not allowing you to pump means risking clogged ducts, mastitis, and other conditions that could force you to miss work. Worried it's not reflecting well on your ambition? Stay a little later, or get a hands-free pumping bra so you can pump while you work.

## INSURANCE, AGAIN

I know. We're almost done, both with this book and with talking about lame logistics like insurance. The last thing you want to worry about while healing and feeding a hangry baby every few hours is hospital bills. Even if your birth is vaginal and uncomplicated, and results in a healthy baby, the tab for intrapartum care (that's just birth—not prenatal or postnatal care or the baby's bill) will still run an average of $30,000. C-sections cost on average 50 percent more. So let's play the broken record one last time in case you glossed over it in trimester zero: Stay on top of your insurance and review your bills.

If you receive an itemized bill, pull the popcorn out and get ready to be entertained. You may find crazy line items like $60 for two ibu-profen, or $500 for skin-to-skin time. As with managing food, this is an excellent project to fork over to your partner to deal with while you heal. Overbilling and clerical errors are not uncommon, especially with complicated medical interactions like birth, so double-check your final tab.

> *Guess how much our epically long birth and five-night stay in the hospital was? Over $110,000! Of that, we paid around $6,000 and insurance paid a little over $30,000. Our insurance is decent, but I wouldn't call it great. Unless your company provides killer benefits, you'll probably end up paying the full yearly out-of-pocket at a minimum. The real entertainment was reliving the insane number of medications, labs, pokes, and prods in line-item for-mat, and seeing how much each "cost." Yet another reminder of how much work our healthcare system still needs.*

## ALWAYS SOMETHING THERE TO REMIND ME

Now, back to a more fun but completely bizarre topic. Chimeras were monstrous fire-breathing mythological beasts with the body of a lion, the head of a goat on one end, and the head of a snake on the other. The term now describes any fictional being made of disparate parts. Which post-pregnancy is you!

Though it sounds more like science fiction, the concept of chi-merism applies to your postpartum body. Even though your baby has vacated your uterus, they left something behind: fetal cells. In fact, if you have an older sibling, some of their cells may be all over your body, too, along with your grandmother's and perhaps even your great-grandmother's.

Georg Schmorl first identified fetal microchimerism,[2] or the presence of fetal cells in a mother's body post-birth, and published the seminal paper on the topic in 1893.[3] These cells are found every-where from the brain, lungs, and heart to the thyroid, breast, and skin.[4] Scientists are still working today to understand their purpose. Their presence is thought to reduce the risk of rheumatoid arthritis,[5] certain autoimmune diseases, and breast cancer, and even to improve wound healing. But we don't really know.

This transfer actually goes both ways.[6] During pregnancy some of the mom's cells cross the placenta and go into the baby's body, too, and are still found there years later. So really, though your baby is no longer literally in your body, and even after they eventually (hopefully) move out of your house, there is a small part of your child that will never leave.

## BIRTH SPACING

This still probably sounds unbelievable, but soon you won't even remember what labor or pregnancy was like.

If you are thinking ahead about your next time around, there are a few things to know about birth spacing. Science currently believes the ideal amount of time for your body to fully normalize between pregnancies is eighteen to twenty-four months, especially if you've had a C-section. Sounds like a long time, sure, but it took nine months to get there, and it takes at least that amount of time to get to your new normal. If, due to age or circumstance, it isn't possible to wait that long, the downsides of starting sooner are increased odds of preterm birth, low birthweight, and even neonatal morbidity.

The best thing to do: Talk to your doctor about your goals, see how your body recovers from this pregnancy and birth, and formulate a plan together.

*I could keep going forever, as there are many deserving topics that didn't make it into these pages. But I'm twelve weeks postpartum, which means my fourth trimester is done, and so is my real-time record of this process. Also, Mr. Baby is ready for a bath and I have a publication deadline.*

*So I'll leave you with this: Enjoy that newborn smell (someone please figure out how to bottle it), and go easy on yourself and all the other parents out there doing the best they can. We're all in this populating and living on the earth thing together, people. Be kind.*

# ACKNOWLEDGMENTS

**T**oni Morrison wrote: "If there's a book that you want to read, but it hasn't been written yet, then you must write it." That sentiment more than any other motivated me to turn my personal journey into the pages you just finished.

As with babies, birthing a book requires a lot of help. I would be nowhere without the wonderful humans who contributed their brains, time, love, and support during our pregnancy journey, and this project. For anyone left out by my hazy postpartum baby brain, I humbly ask for your forgiveness.

First, to my team at Simon and Schuster, thank you for patiently letting me do the somewhat insane thing of writing this book in real time, especially when I had a newborn around. Theresa DiMasi, thanks for believing I had this book in me the first time we spoke, and for being awesome at every step. Anja Schmidt for all the encouragement and enthusiasm along the way. Kate Davids, your investigative skills and inquisitive mind contributed so much to these pages, and you have my eternal gratitude. Polly Watson, thank you for making me repeatedly LOL with the copyedit and reminding me that all toads are frogs, but not all frogs are toads. Nancy Tonik, you and your team dealt with my many edits and perfectionist tendencies, and for that you deserve a trophy. And to my editor, Emily Carleton, thanks for coaching me through it as a first-time author.

To the marvelous Jane van Dis, thanks for sharing your many years of obstetrical expertise and editorial prowess. Your cheerleading and brainstorming during this project made it so much better.

Many smart people allowed me to borrow their minds and many years of experience during the writing of this book. I am so grateful for their contributions not only to these pages but also to my own pregnancy: Amy Brandon, MD; Alexandra Brown, founder of the Muscle Butter; Alex Capano, DNP, CRNP, FNP-BC; Carine Carmy, founder of Origin; Heather Charmatz, SF Birth Doula; Michaela Cruze, prenatal and postnatal personal trainer; Ciara Devereux, marriage and family therapist, MA; Meleah Ekstrand, Inner Strength Birth; Mary Beth Ferrante, founder of Live.Work.Lead; Valerie Flaherman, MD; Martina Fogt, MPT, women's health and pelvic floor specialist; Myles Lewis, CrossFit Avalanche; Aliza Marogy, ND, founder of Inessa Wellness; Mercedes Samudio, founder of Shame-Proof Parenting; Sara Stieg, founder of Nest Acupuncture; Jackie Stone, MD; Kendra Tolbert, MS, RDN, CDN, LD, RYT, Cert AT; Nina Wilson, CNM, IBCLC; Danika Wynn, CNM, IBCLC. A special thanks also to Kalliope White at Maven for facilitating many of these interviews.

Kate Ryder, your friendship contributed greatly to both my personal experience and so many parts of this book. Thanks for your fearlessness, and for letting me tag along as part of the Maven family.

Dondeena Bradley, thank you for doing that magical connection thing you do, and for helping me believe I should take on this project.

Deepest thanks to the generous humans who tolerated pregnancy trivia over dinner and mocktails, provided parenting pro tips, design consultations, and publishing advice, took waddles to Crissy Field, and went above and beyond in the friendship department: Aliza Marogy, Amy Lockwood, Andrew and Nicole Weiss, Arian Van de Carr, Ashlee Adams, Aza Raskin, Clare Wylie, Jenn Hirsch, Kieran Kieckhefer, Kim Lembo, Kim Taylor, Linda Avey, Michael Brooks, Morgan Chaney,

Scott Gallacher, Seychelle Engelhard, Stacy Stokes, Susan Coelius Keplinger, and Victoria Graham.

Special thanks to Ryan Panchadsaram and Suhasini Chandramouli for the glut of books, advice, check-ins, and encouragement on all sides of this journey. Mr. Baby looks forward to a lifetime of playdates with Ansel.

Christy Habetz, it was your strength and grace I channeled in every challenging moment.

Megan Miller, my baby mage, I still think *you* should have written this book (though I hope I did your advice credit).

Lisa Forster and Kathy Chan, thanks for being my first pregnant readers and dear friends for so many years.

Anne Devereux-Mills, Ciara Devereux, and Lauren Burns: those long sixteen months would have been impossible to nagivate without your love and support. Lauren, thank you for being my sounding board and letting me pepper you with constant requests for feedback. Ciara, your wisdom influenced so many of the therapy sections of this book. And, Anne, from coral foot to the D&C, you have been there through it all and I don't know what I would do without you, today and always. Nick, Mr. Baby, and I are so very lucky to call the three of you family.

Miracle Monica, you cared for (and taught) Nick and me just as much as Mr. Baby. We can't wait to do it with you all over again.

To our families, thank you for all the support in this process, and for embracing your roles as aunts, uncles, grandparents, and cousins with such enthusiasm. Mr. Baby is a lucky dude. Special thanks to my parents for bringing me up to believe that there was nothing I couldn't do, like write this book.

Magnus, you're a dog and can't read this. But I'm grateful for all the hours you faithfully spent sleeping by my feet while I was large and pregnant and writing this book, and even now editing these final pages. You're a very good boy.

Nick, my hype man and number one cheerleader, you let me bore you with random pregnancy facts, provided the dude's perspective, named this book, helped with edits, kept me going during the rough periods, and, most of all, made me laugh every single day—and still do. I love you so much.

And finally, to my greatest creation, Mr. Baby: Thank you for making me a mom.

# NOTES

## PREFACE

1  "How Common Is Infertility?" Eunice Kennedy Shriver National Institute of Child Health and Human Development, accessed August 8, 2019, https://www.nichd.nih.gov/health/topics/infertility/conditioninfo/common.

2. Krissi Danielsson, "Making Sense of Miscarriage Statistics," Verywell Family, March 15, 2019, accessed August 8, 2019, https://www.verywellfamily.com/making-sense-of-miscarriage-statistics-2371721.

3. "Improving Maternal Mental Health Care," California Health Care Foundation, last modified May 23, 2019, https://www.chcf.org/project/improving-treatment-of-maternal-mental-health/.

4. T. J. Mathews and B. E. Hamilton, "Mean Age of Mother, 1970–2000," *National Vital Statistics Reports* 51, no. 1 (December 11, 2002).

5. Joyce A. Martin et al., "Births: Final Data for 2017," *National Vital Statistics Reports* 67, no. 8 (November 7, 2018).

6. Quoctrung Bui and Claire Cain Miller, "The Age That Women Have Babies: How a Gap Divides America," *New York Times*, August 4, 2018, accessed August 8, 2019, https://www.nytimes.com/interactive/2018/08/04/upshot/up-birth-age-gap.html?mtrref=undefined&gwh=89C31420B8695A960AE91DBB2EEAFE47&gwt=pay&assetType=REGIWALL.

7. Zoë Slote Morris, Steven Wooding, and Jonathan Grant, "The Answer Is 17 Years, What Is the Question: Understanding Time Lags in Translational Research," *Journal of the Royal Society of Medicine* 104, no. 12 (December 2011), accessed August 8, 2019, https://doi.org/10.1258/jrsm.2011.110180.

8. Anne Drapkin Lyerly and Ruth R. Faden, "Mothers Matter: Ethics and Research during Pregnancy," *American Medical Association Journal of Ethics* 15, no. 9 (September 2013), accessed August 8, 2019, https://journalofethics.ama-assn.org/article/mothers-matter-ethics -and-research-during-pregnancy/2013-09.

# TRIMESTER ZERO

1. Naina Kumar and Amit Kant Singh, "Trends of Male Factor Infertility, an Important Cause of Infertility: A Review of Literature," *Journal of Human Reproductive Sciences* 8, no. 4 (2015): 191–96, doi:10.4103/0974-1208.170370.

## *Get Your Bodies and Lives Ready*

1. Jill E. Yavorsky et al., "The Production of Inequality: The Gender Division of Labor Across the Transition to Parenthood," *Journal of Marriage and the Family* 77, no. 3 (June 2015): 662–79, https://doi .org/10.1111/jomf.12189.
2. Susan K. Murphy et al., "Cannabinoid Exposure and Altered DNA Methylation in Rat and Human Sperm," *Epigenetics* 13, no. 12 (December 2018): 1208–21, https://doi.org/10.1080/15592294.2018.1554521.
3. "About Chronic Diseases," Centers for Disease Control and Prevention, accessed June 22, 2019, https://www.cdc.gov/chronicdisease/about /index.htm.
4. "Frequently Asked Questions: Pregnancy; Carrier Screening," American College of Obstetricians and Gynecologists, December 2018, https:// www.acog.org/Patients/FAQs/Carrier-Screening.
5. Jonatan Axelsson et al., "Association Between Paternal Smoking at the Time of Pregnancy and the Semen Quality in Sons," *PLoS ONE* 13, no. 11 (November 2018): e0207221, https://doi.org/10.1371/journal .pone.0207221.
6. Bob Weinhold, "Epigenetics: The Science of Change," *Environmental Health Perspectives* 114, no. 3 (March 2006): A160–67, https://doi .org/10.1289/ehp.114-a160.
7. Hannah Blencowe et al., "Folic Acid to Reduce Neonatal Mortality from Neural Tube Disorders," *International Journal of Epidemiology* 39, Supplement 1 (April 2010): i110–21, https://doi.org/10.1093/ije /dyq028.

8.  Janet M. Catov et al., "Periconceptional Multivitamin Use and Risk of Preterm or Small-for-Gestational-Age Births in the Danish National Birth Cohort," *American Journal of Clinical Nutrition* 94, no. 3 (September 2011): 906–12, https://doi.org/10.3945/ajcn.111.012393.

9.  Wikipedia, s.v. "Lucy Wills," accessed June 22, 2019, https://en.wikipedia.org/wiki/Lucy_Wills.

10. "MTHFR Gene," National Institutes of Health Genetics Home Reference, accessed June 22, 2019, https://ghr.nlm.nih.gov/gene/MTHFR.

11. "Data & Statistics on Birth Defects," Centers for Disease Control and Prevention, accessed June 22, 2019, https://www.cdc.gov/ncbddd/birthdefects/data.html.

12. "Data & Statistics on Zika and Pregnancy," Centers for Disease Control and Prevention, accessed June 22, 2019, https://www.cdc.gov/pregnancy/zika/data/.

13. "A Typical American Birth Costs as Much as Delivering a Royal Baby," *Economist*, April 23, 2018, https://www.economist.com/graphic-detail/2018/04/23/a-typical-american-birth-costs-as-much-as-delivering-a-royal-baby.

14. "Center for Nutrition Policy and Promotion," US Department of Agriculture Food and Nutrition Service, accessed June 22, 2019, https://www.fns.usda.gov/cnpp/center-nutrition-policy-and-promotion.

15. "This Is How Much Child Care Costs in 2019," Care.com, July 15, 2019, https://www.care.com/c/stories/2423/how-much-does-child-care-cost/.

16. David G. Blanchflower and Andrew E. Clark, "Children, Unhappiness, and Family Finances: Evidence from One Million Europeans," NBER Working Paper No. 25597, National Bureau of Economic Research, Cambridge, MA, February 2019, https://www.nber.org/papers/w25597.

17. Mark DeWolf, "12 Stats About Working Women," US *Department of Labor Blog*, March 1, 2017, https://blog.dol.gov/2017/03/01/12-stats-about-working-women.

18. Laura Addati, Naomi Cassirer, and Katherine Gilchrist, *Maternity and Paternity at Work: Law and Practice Across the World* (Geneva, Switzerland: International Labour Office, 2014), http://www.ilo.org/wcmsp5/groups/public/---dgreports/---dcomm/---publ/documents/publication/wcms_242615.pdf.

19. Trish Stroman et al., "Why Paid Family Leave Is Good Business," BCG Henderson Institute, February 7, 2017, https://www.bcg.com/publications/2017/human-resources-people-organization-why-paid-family-leave-is-good-business.aspx.

20. "Wage and Hour Division: FMLA Frequently Asked Questions," US Department of Labor, accessed June 22, 2019, https://www.dol.gov /whd/fmla/fmla-faqs.htm.

### *Your Care Team Fantasy Draft*

1. Richard W. Wertz, Dorothy C. Wertz, and Barbara Howe, *Lying-In: A History of Childbirth in America* (New Haven, CT: Yale University Press, 1989).

2. "The History of Chicago Lying-In Hospital," Chicago Lying-In Hospital, accessed June 22, 2019, https://chicagolyinginboard.uchicago .edu/chicago-lying-in-history/.

3. Judith W. Leavitt, "Joseph B. DeLee and the Practice of Preventive Obstetrics," *American Journal of Public Health* 78, no. 10 (October 1988): 1353–60, https://ajph.aphapublications.org/doi/pdf/10.2105/AJP H.78.10.1353.

4. "The US Needs More Midwives for Better Maternity Care," *Scientific American*, February 1, 2019, https://www.scientificamerican.com/article /the-u-s-needs-more-midwives-for-better-maternity-care/.

5. "Committee Opinion on Planned Home Births," American College of Obstetricians and Gynecologists, April 2017, https://www.acog .org/Clinical-Guidance-and-Publications/Committee-Opinions /Committee-on-Obstetric-Practice/Planned-Home-Birth.

6. Meghan A. Bohren et al., "Continuous Support for Women During Childbirth," *Cochrane Database of Systematic Reviews*, July 6, 2017, https://doi.org/10.1002/14651858.CD003766.pub6.

7. Katy Backes Kozhimannil et al., "Doula Care, Birth Outcomes, and Costs Among Medicaid Beneficiaries," *American Journal of Public Health* 103, no. 4 (2013): e113–21, https://doi.org/10.2105/AJPH.2012 .301201.

8. M. Armour et al., "Acupuncture and Acupressure for Premenstrual Syndrome," *Cochrane Database of Systematic Reviews*, August 14, 2018, https://doi.org/10.1002/14651858.CD005290.pub2.

9. Ibid.

10. S. D. Liddle and V. Pennick, "Interventions for Preventing and Treating Low-Back and Pelvic Pain During Pregnancy," *Cochrane Database of Systematic Reviews*, September 30, 2015, https://doi.org /10.1002/14651858.CD001139.pub4.

11. Tiffany Field, "Pregnancy and Labor Massage," *Expert Review of Obstetrics & Gynecology* 5, no. 2 (January 2014): 177–81, https://doi .org/10.1586/eog.10.12.

12. Seewon Ryu, "History of Telemedicine: Evolution, Context, and Transformation," *Healthcare Informatics Research* 16, no. 1 (March 2010): 65–66, https://doi.org/10.4258/hir.2010.16.1.65.

13. F. Benvenuti et al., "Reeducative Treatment of Female Genuine Stress Incontinence," *American Journal of Physical Medicine* 66, no. 4 (August 1987): 155–68, https://www.ncbi.nlm.nih.gov/pubmed/3674220.

14. S. J. Woodley et al., "Pelvic Floor Muscle Training for Prevention and Treatment of Urinary and Faecal Incontinence in Antenatal and Postnatal Women," *Cochrane Database of Systematic Reviews*, December 22, 2017, https://doi.org/10.1002/14651858.CD007471.pub3.

15. Y. Du et al., "The Effect of Antenatal Pelvic Floor Muscle Training on Labor and Delivery Outcomes: A Systematic Review with Meta-Analysis," *International Urogynecology Journal* 26, no. 10 (October 2015): 1415–27, https://doi.org/10.1007/s00192-015-2654-4.

## *Making a Baby*

1. "First Births to Older Women Continue to Rise," Centers for Disease Control and Prevention, last modified May 2014, https://www.cdc.gov/nchs/products/databriefs/db152.htm.

2. A. Z. Steiner et al., "Association Between Biomarkers of Ovarian Reserve and Infertility Among Older Women of Reproductive Age," *Journal of the American Medical Association* 318, no. 14 (2017): 1367–76, https://doi.org/10.1001/jama.2017.14588.

3. Holly Eagleson, "Your Chances of Getting Pregnant at Every Age," *Parents*, last modified June 22, 2019, https://www.parents.com/getting-pregnant/trying-to-conceive/up-your-chances-of-getting-pregnant-at-every-age/.

4. *National Public Health Action Plan for the Detection, Prevention, and Management of Infertility* (Atlanta: Centers for Disease Control and Prevention, 2014), https://www.cdc.gov/reproductivehealth/infertility/pdf/drh_nap_final_508.pdf.

5. "Trying to Conceive," Office on Women's Health, last updated June 6, 2018, https://www.womenshealth.gov/pregnancy/you-get-pregnant/trying-conceive.

6. S. S. Suarez and A. A. Pacey, "Sperm Transport in the Female Reproductive Tract," *Human Reproduction Update* 12, no. 1 (January–February 2006): 23–37, https://doi.org/10.1093/humupd/dmi047.

7. John Jude Kweku Annan et al., "Biochemical Pregnancy During Assisted Conception: A Little Bit Pregnant," *Journal of Clinical Medicine Research* 5, no. 4 (August 2013): 269–74, https://doi.org/10.4021/jocmr1008w.

## *If Things Get Bumpy*

1.  Lauren M. Rossen, Katherine A. Ahrens, and Amy M. Branum, "Trends in Risk of Pregnancy Loss Among US Women, 1990–2011," *Paediatric and Perinatal Epidemiology* 32, no. 1 (January 2018): 19–29, doi.org/10.1111/ppe.12417.

2.  A. J. Wilcox et al., "Incidence of Early Loss of Pregnancy," *New England Journal of Medicine,* no. 319 (July 1988): 189–94, https://doi.org/10.1056/nejm198807283190401

3.  Alexandra C. Sundermann et al., "Alcohol Use in Pregnancy and Miscarriage: A Systematic Review and Meta-Analysis," *Alcoholism Clinical and Experimental Research* 43, no. 8 (August 2019): 1606–16, https://doi.org/10.1111/acer.14124.

4.  "Multiple Miscarriage," National Infertility Association, accessed June 24, 2019, https://resolve.org/infertility-101/medical-conditions/multiple-miscarriage/.

5.  "Infertility FAQs," Centers for Disease Control and Prevention, accessed June 24, 2019, https://www.cdc.gov/reproductivehealth/infertility/index.htm.

6.  Naina Kumar and Amit Kant Singh, "Trends of Male Factor Infertility, an Important Cause of Infertility: A Review of Literature," *Journal of Human Reproductive Sciences* 8, no. 4 (October–December 2015): 191–96, https://doi.org/10.4103/0974-1208.170370.

7.  Hagai Levine et al., "Temporal Trends in Sperm Count: A Systematic Review and Meta-regression Analysis," *Human Reproduction* 23, no. 6 (November–December 2017): 646–59, https://doi.org/10.1093/humupd/dmx022.

8.  Ibid.

9.  Daniel Noah Halpern, "Sperm Count Zero," *GQ*, September 4, 2018, https://www.gq.com/story/sperm-count-zero.

10. European Society of Human Reproduction and Embryology, "More than 8 Million Babies Born from IVF Since the World's First in 1978: European IVF Pregnancy Rates Now Steady at Around 36 Percent, According to ESHRE Monitoring," *ScienceDaily*, July 3, 2018, https://www.sciencedaily.com/releases/2018/07/180703084127.htm.

# THE FIRST TRIMESTER

1. Paul W. Sherman and Samuel M. Flaman, "Morning Sickness: A Mechanism for Protecting Mother and Embryo," *Quarterly Review of Biology* 75, no. 2 (June 2000), https://pdfs.semanticscholar.org/e289/e676e163acbd56d1943a848f1a4ee45d1b45.pdf.

## Pregnancy FAQ, Lightning Round

1. H. T. Duong et al., "Maternal Use of Hot Tub and Major Structural Birth Defects," *Birth Defects Research Part A: Clinical and Molecular Teratology* 91, no. 9 (September 2011): 836–41, https://doi.org/10.1002/bdra.20831.
2. Elseline Hoekzema et al., "Pregnancy Leads to Long-Lasting Changes in Human Brain Structure," *Nature America* 20, no. 2 (February 2017): 287–96, https://doi.org/10.1038/nn.4458.
3. John Askling et al., "Sickness in Pregnancy and Sex of Child," *Lancet* 354, no. 9195 (December 11, 1999), https://doi.org/10.1016/S0140-6736(99)04239-7.
4. J. L. Jones et al., "Risk Factors for Toxoplasma Gondii Infection in the United States," *Clinical Infectious Diseases* 49, no. 6 (September 2009): 878–84, https://doi.org/10.1086/605433.
5. A. J. C. Cook et al., "Sources of Toxoplasma Infection in Pregnant Women; European Multicentre Case-Control Study," *BMJ* 321, no. 7254 (July 2000): 142–47, doi.org/10.1136/bmj.321.7254.142.

## The Pregnancy Commandments

1. Sarah K. Griffiths and Jeremy P. Campbell, "Placental Structure, Function and Drug Transfer," *Continuing Education in Anaesthesia Critical Care & Pain* 15, no. 2 (April 2015): 84–89, https://doi.org/10.1093/bjaceaccp/mku013.
2. "Appendix D: Teratogens/Prenatal Substance Abuse," in *Understanding Genetics: A District of Columbia Guide for Patients and Health Professionals* (Washington, DC: Genetic Alliance, 2010), https://www.ncbi.nlm.nih.gov/books/NBK132140/.
3. P. A. May et al., "Prevalence of Fetal Alcohol Spectrum Disorders in 4 US Communities," *Journal of the American Medical Association* 319, no. 5 (February 2018): 474–82, https://doi.org/10.1001/jama.2017.21896.
4. "Tobacco, Alcohol, Drugs, and Pregnancy," American College of Obstetricians and Gynecologists, February 2019, https://www.acog.org/Patients/FAQs/Tobacco-Alcohol-Drugs-and-Pregnancy#fetal.

5.   Wayne B. Conover, Thomas C. Key, and Robert Resnik, "Maternal Cardiovascular Response to Caffeine Infusion in the Pregnant Ewe," *American Journal of Obstetrics & Gynecology* 145, no. 5 (March 1983): 534–38, https://doi.org/10.1016/0002-9378(83)91191-2.

6.   "Substance Use During Pregnancy," Centers for Disease Control and Prevention, accessed June 24, 2019, https://www.cdc.gov/reproductive health/maternalinfanthealth/substance-abuse/substance-abuse-during -pregnancy.htm.

7.   Tatiana M. Anderson et al., "Maternal Smoking Before and During Pregnancy and the Risk of Sudden Unexpected Infant Death," *Pediatrics* 143, no. 4 (April 2019), https://doi.org/10.1542/peds.2018-3325.

8.   "Marijuana and Cancer," American Cancer Society, accessed June 21, 2019, https://www.cancer.org/treatment/treatments-and-side-effects /complementary-and-alternative-medicine/marijuana-and-cancer .html.

9.   Susan K. Murphy et al., "Cannabinoid Exposure and Altered DNA Methylation in Rat and Human Sperm," *Epigenetics* 13, no. 12 (December 2018): 1208–21, https://doi.org/10.1080/15592294.2018.1 554521.

10.   J. K. Gunn et al., "Prenatal Exposure to Cannabis and Maternal and Child Health Outcomes: A Systematic Review and Meta-analysis," *BMJ Open* 6, no. 4 (April 2016), https://doi.org/10.1136/bmj open-2015-009986.

11.   Marcel O. Bonn-Miller et al., "Labeling Accuracy of Cannabidiol Extracts Sold Online," *Journal of the American Medical Association* 318, no. 17 (November 2017): 1708–9, https://doi.org/10.1001/jama .2017.11909.

12.   M. K. Trivedi et al., "A Review of the Safety of Cosmetic Procedures During Pregnancy and Lactation," *International Journal of Women's Dermatology* 3, no.1 (February 2017): 6–10, https://doi.org/10.1016/j .ijwd.2017.01.005.

13.   Pina Bozzo et al., "Safety of Skin Care Products During Pregnancy," *Canadian Family Physician* 57, no. 6 (June 2011): 665–67.

14.   Elise Labonte-Lemoyne, Daniel Curnier, and Dave Ellemberg, "Exercise During Pregnancy Enhances Cerebral Maturation in the Newborn: A Randomized Controlled Trial," *Journal of Clinical and Experimental Neuropsychology* 39, no. 4 (2017): 347–54, https://doi.org /10.1080/13803395.2016.1227427.

15.   M. Bahls et al., "Mothers' Exercise During Pregnancy Programmes Vasomotor Function in Adult Offspring," *Experimental Physiology* 99,

no. 1 (January 2014): 205–19, https://doi.org/10.1113/expphysiol.2013 .0759978.

16.  "Weight Gain During Pregnancy," American College of Obstetricians and Gynecologists, January 2013, https://www.acog.org/Clinical-Guidance-and -Publications/Committee-Opinions/Committee-on-Obstetric-Practice /Weight-Gain-During-Pregnancy.

## To Test, or Not to Test?

1.  Malcolm Nicolson and John E. E. Fleming, *Imaging and Imagining the Fetus: The Development of Obstetric Ultrasound* (Baltimore: Johns Hopkins University Press, 2013), https://muse.jhu.edu/.

2.  "Ultrasound Imaging," US Food & Drug Administration, last modi- fied August 29, 2018, https://www.fda.gov/radiation-emitting-products /medical-imaging/ultrasound-imaging.

3.  "First Trimester Screening," Mayo Clinic, accessed July 8, 2019, https://www.mayoclinic.org/tests-procedures/first-trimester-screening /about/pac-20394169.

4.  B. Brambati and G. Simoni, "Diagnosis of Fetal Trisomy 21 in First Trimester," *Lancet* 321, no. 8324 (March 12, 1983): 586, doi:10.1016 /S0140-6736(83)92831-3.

5.  "Amniocentesis," Science Museum, accessed July 8, 2019, http:// broughttolife,sciencemuseum.org.uk/broughttolife/techniques/amni ocentesis.

6.  "Amniocentesis," Mayo Clinic, accessed July 8, 2019, https://www .mayoclinic.org/tests-procedures/amniocentesis/about/pac-20392 914.

7.  "Rh Factor Blood Test," Mayo Clinic, accessed July 8, 2019, https:// www.mayoclinic.org/tests-procedures/rh-factor/about/pac-20394960.

8.  "Gestational Diabetes," Centers for Disease Control and Prevention, accessed July 8, 2019, https://www.cdc.gov/diabetes/basics/gestational .html.

9.  "Group B Strep," Centers for Disease Control and Prevention, accessed July 8, 2019, https://www.cdc.gov/groupbstrep/.

10.  Hiromi Nagase et al., "Fetal outcome of trisomy 18 diagnosed after 22 weeks of gestation: Experience of 123 cases at a single perinatal center," *Congenital Abnormalities* 56, no. 1 (January 2016): 35–40, https://doi.org/10.1111/cga.12118.

# THE SECOND TRIMESTER

## What Do I Actually Need to Buy?

1. Lindsay Manning, "A Brief History of Maternity Clothes," *Huffington Post*, last modified February 2009, https://www.huffpost.com /entry/a-brief-history-of-matern_b_156618.
2. Helena Lee, "Why Finnish Babies Sleep in Cardboard Boxes," *BBC News*, June 4, 2013, https://www.bbc.com/news/magazine-22751415.
3. "Finland's Low Infant Mortality Has Multiple Contributing Factors," *Terveyden Ja Hyvinvoinnin Laitos* (blog), January 27, 2017, https://blogi. thl.fi/finlands-low-infant-mortality-has-multiple-contributing-factors/.

## Let's Get Physical

1. Caitlin Thurber et al., "Extreme Events Reveal an Alimentary Limit on Sustained Maximal Human Energy Expenditure," *Science Advances* 5, no. 6 (June 2019), https://doi.org/10.1126/sciadv.aaw0341.
2. M. M. Beckmann and O. M. Stock, "Antenatal Perineal Massage for Reducing Perineal Trauma," *Cochrane Database of Systematic Reviews*, April 30, 2013, doi:10.1002/14651858.CD005123.pub3.
3. Jessica Keller et al., "Diastasis Recti Abdominis: A Survey of Women's Health Specialists for Current Physical Therapy Clinical Practice for Postpartum Women," *Journal of Women's Health Physical Therapy* 36, no. 3 (September–December 2012): 131–42, https://doi.org/10.1097 /JWH.0b013e318276f35f.
4. J. B. Sperstad et al., "Diastasis Recti Abdominis During Pregnancy and 12 Months After Childbirth: Prevalence, Risk Factors and Report of Lumbopelvic Pain," *British Journal of Sports Medicine* 50, no. 17 (September 2016): 1092–96, https://bjsm.bmj.com/content /50/17/1092.

## It's Not a Birth Plan—It's Preferences

1. Josephine M. Green and Helen A. Baston, "Feeling in Control During Labor: Concepts, Correlates, and Consequences," *Birth* 30, no. 4 (January 2004): 235–47, https://doi.org/10.1046/j.1523-536X.2003.00253.x.
2. O. Moscucci, "Holistic Obstetrics: The Origins of 'Natural Childbirth' in Britain," *Postgraduate Medical Journal* 79, no. 929 (March 2003): 168–73, https://pmj.bmj.com/content/79/929/168.

3. Michelle J. K. Osterman and Joyce A. Martin, "Epidural and Spinal Anesthesia Use During Labor: 27-State Reporting Area, 2008," *National Vital Statistics Reports* 59, no. 5 (April 6, 2011), https://www.cdc.gov/nchs/data/nvsr/nvsr59/nvsr59_05.pdf.

4. "Anesthesia and Queen Victoria," UCLA Department of Epidemiology, accessed June 22, 2019, https://www.ph.ucla.edu/epi/snow/victoria.html.

5. Yiska Loewenberg-Weisband et al., "Epidural Analgesia and Severe Perineal Tears: A Literature Review and Large Cohort Study," *Journal of Maternal-Fetal & Neonatal Medicine* 27, no. 18 (March 2014): 1864–69, https://www.doi.org/10.3109/14767058.2014.889113.

6. Nathan Hitzeman and Shannon Chin, "Epidural Analgesia for Labor Pain," *American Family Physician* 86, no. 3 (August 2012): 241–42, https://www.aafp.org/afp/2012/0801/p241.html.

7. Cynthia A. French, Xiaomei Cong, and Keun Sam Chung, "Labor Epidural Analgesia and Breastfeeding: A Systematic Review," *Journal of Human Lactation* 32, no. 3 (August 2016): 507–20, https://doi.org/10.1177/0890334415623779.

8. Lissa Borup et al., "Acupuncture as Pain Relief During Delivery: A Randomized Controlled Trial," *Birth* 36, no. 1 (March 2009): 5–12, https://doi.org/10.1111/j.1523-536X.2008.00290.x.

9. Eun Hee Cho et al., "The Effects of Aromatherapy on Intensive Care Unit Patients' Stress and Sleep Quality: A Nonrandomised Controlled Trial," *Evidence-Based Complementary and Alternative Medicine* (December 2017), https://doi.org/10.1155/2017/2856592.

10. Juli Reynolds et al., "Using Aromatherapy in the Clinical Setting: Making Sense of Scents," *American Nurse Today* 13, no. 6 (June 2018), https://www.americannursetoday.com/aromatherapy-clinical-setting/.

11. S. Downe et al., "Self-Hypnosis for Intrapartum Pain Management in Pregnant Nulliparous Women: A Randomised Controlled Trial of Clinical Effectiveness," *BJOG* 122, no. 9 (August 2015): 1226–34, https://doi.org/10.1111/1471-0528.13433.

12. C. A. Smith et al., "Massage, Reflexology and Other Manual Methods for Pain Management in Labour," *Cochrane Database of Systematic Reviews*, March 28, 2018, https://doi.org/10.1002/14651858.CD009290.pub3.

13. E. R. Cluett and A. Cuthbert, "Immersion in Water During Labour and Birth," *Cochrane Database of Systematic Reviews*, May 16, 2018, https://doi.org/10.1002/14651858.CD000111.pub4.

14. "The Effect of TENS for Pain Relief in Labor," Cochrane

Complementary Medicine, accessed June 22, 2019, https://cam .cochrane.org/effect-tens-pain-relief-labor.

15. "83 Percent Say Measles Vaccine Is Safe for Healthy Children," Pew Research Center, February 9, 2015, https://www.people-press .org/2015/02/09/83-percent-say-measles-vaccine-is-safe-for-healthy -children/.

16. Jennie Schoeppe et al., "The Immunity Community: A Community Engagement Strategy for Reducing Vaccine Hesitancy," *Health Promotion Practice* 18, no. 5 (September 2017): 654–61, https://doi .org/10.1177/1524839917697303.

17. "Benefits from Immunization During the Vaccines for Children Program Era—1994–2013," Centers for Disease Control and Prevention, last modified April 25, 2014, https://www.cdc.gov/mmwr/preview/mmwrhtml /mm6316a4.htm.

18. "Ten Threats to Global Health in 2019," World Health Association, accessed June 22, 2019, https://www.who.int/emergencies/ten-threats -to-global-health-in-2019.

19. Roger Collier, "Circumcision Indecision: The Ongoing Saga of the World's Most Popular Surgery," *Canadian Medical Association Journal* 183, no. 17 (November 2011): 1961–62, https://doi.org/10.1503 /cmaj.109-4021.

20. Geoffrey D. Hart-Cooper et al., "Circumcision of Privately Insured Males Aged 0 to 18 Years in the United States," *Pediatrics* 134, no. 5 (November 2014): 950–56, https://doi.org/10.1542/peds.2014-1007.

21. Helen A. Weiss et al., "Complications of Circumcision in Male Neonates, Infants and Children: A Systematic Review," *BMC Urology* 10, no. 2 (February 2010), https://doi.org/10.1186/1471-2490-10-2.

22. Brian J. Morris et al., "Does Male Circumcision Affect Sexual Function, Sensitivity, or Satisfaction?—A Systematic Review," *Journal of Sexual Medicine* 10, no. 11 (August 2013): 2644–57, https://www .jsm.jsexmed.org/article/S1743-6095(15)30172-7/.

23. John N. Krieger et al., "Adult Male Circumcision: Effects on Sexual Function and Sexual Satisfaction in Kisumu, Kenya," *Journal of Sexual Medicine* 5, no. 11 (November 2008): 2610–22, https://doi .org/10.1111/j.1743-6109.2008.00979.x.

24. "Cord Blood Banking," American College of Obstetricians and Gynecologists, February 2016, https://www.acog.org/Patients/FAQs /Cord-Blood-Banking.

25. "Delayed Umbilical Cord Clamping Position Statement," American College of Nurse-Midwives, 2014, http://www.midwife.org/ACNM

/files/ACNMLibraryData/UPLOADFILENAME/000000000290
/Delayed-Umbilical-Cord-Clamping-May-2014.pdf.

26. S. J. McDonald, "Effect of Timing of Umbilical Cord Clamping of Term Infants on Maternal and Neonatal Outcomes," *Cochrane Database of Systematic Reviews*, July 11, 2013, https://doi.org/10.1002 /14651858.CD004074.pub3.

27. Anup C. Katheria et al., "Umbilical Cord Milking Versus Delayed Cord Clamping in Preterm Infants," *Pediatrics* 136, no. 1 (July 2015), 61–69, https://doi.org/10.1542/peds.2015-0368.

28. L. K. Gryder et al., "Effects of Human Maternal Placentophagy on Maternal Postpartum Iron Status: A Randomized, Double-Blind, Placebo-Controlled Pilot Study," *Journal of Midwifery & Women's Health* 62, no. 1 (January 2017): 68–79, https://doi.org/10.1111 /jmwh.12549.

29. G. L. Buser et al., "Notes from the Field: Late-Onset Infant Group B Streptococcus Infection Associated with Maternal Consumption of Capsules Containing Dehydrated Placenta—Oregon," *Morbidity and Mortality Weekly Report* 66, no. 25 (June 30, 2017): 677–78, https:// doi.org/http://dx.doi.org/10.15585/mmwr.mm6625a.

30. Alexandra C. Sundermann et al., "Alcohol Use in Pregnancy and Miscarriage: A Systematic Review and Meta-Analysis," *Alcoholism Clinical & Experimental Research* 43, no. 8 (August 2019): 1606–16, https://doi.org/10.1111/acer.14124.

31. S. H. Jaafar, J. J. Ho, and K. S. Lee, "Rooming-In for New Mother and Infant Versus Separate Care for Increasing the Duration of Breastfeeding," *Cochrane Database of Systematic Reviews*, August 26, 2016, https://doi.org/10.1002/14651858.CD006641.pub3.

# THE THIRD TRIMESTER

## *The Big Event*

1. Manjeet Singh Bhatia and Anurag Jhanjee, "Tokophobia: A Dread of Pregnancy," *Industrial Psychiatry Journal* 21, no. 2 (July–December 2012): 158–59, https://doi.org/10.4103/0972-6748.119649.

2. Simona Labor and Simon Maguire, "The Pain of Labour," *Reviews in Pain* 2, no. 2 (December 2008): 15–19, https://doi.org /10.1177/204946370800200205.

3. Amina Z. Khambalia et al., "Predicting Date of Birth and Examining

the Best Time to Date a Pregnancy," *International Journal of Gynecology & Obstetrics* 123, no. 2 (November 2013): 105–9, https://doi.org/10.1016/j.ijgo.2013.05.007.

4. Anna S. Oberg et al., "Maternal and Fetal Genetic Contributions to Postterm Birth: Familial Clustering in a Population-Based Sample of 475,429 Swedish Births," *American Journal of Epidemiology* 177, no. 6 (March 15, 2013): 531–37, https://doi.org/10.1093/aje/kws244.

5. Gordon C. S. Smith, "Use of Time to Event Analysis to Estimate the Normal Duration of Human Pregnancy," *Human Reproduction* 16, no. 7 (July 2001): 1497–1500, doi.org/10.1093/humrep/16.7.1497.

6. "If Your Baby Is Breech," American College of Obstetricians and Gynecologists, last modified January 2019, https://www.acog.org/Patients/FAQs/If-Your-Baby-Is-Breech.

7. M. Smith et al., "External Cephalic Version in Cases of Breech Presentation: Renaissance of a Well-Known Procedure?" *Gynecological Obstetric Rundsch* 49, no. 1 (2009): 29–34, https://doi.org/10.1159/000184443.

8. Terry C. Harper et al., "A Randomized Controlled Trial of Acupuncture for Initiation of Labor in Nulliparous Women," *Journal of Maternal-Fetal & Neonatal Medicine* 19, no. 8 (2006): 465–70, https://doi.org/10.1080/14767050600730740.

9. Caroline A. Smith, M. Armour, and H. G. Dahle, "Acupuncture or Acupressure for Induction of Labour," *Cochrane Database of Systematic Reviews*, October 17, 2017, https://doi.org/10.1002/14651858.CD002962.pub4.

10. O. Al-Kuran et al., "The Effect of Late Pregnancy Consumption of Date Fruit on Labour and Delivery," *Journal of Obstetrics and Gynaecology* 31, no. 1 (January 2011): 29–31, https://doi.org/10.3109/01443615.2010.522267.

11. Nuguelis Razali et al., "Date Fruit Consumption at Term: Effect on Length of Gestation, Labour and Delivery," *Journal of Obstetrics and Gynaecology* 37, no. 5 (July 2017): 595–600, https://doi.org/10.1080/01443615.2017.1283304.

12. Aaron B. Caughey et al., *Maternal and Neonatal Outcomes of Elective Induction of Labor* (Rockville, MD: Agency for Healthcare Research and Quality, 2009), https://www.ncbi.nlm.nih.gov/books/NBK38683/.

13. William A. Grobman et al., "Labor Induction Versus Expectant Management in Low-Risk Nulliparous Women," *New England Journal of Medicine*, no. 379 (August 2018): 513–23, https://doi.org/10.1056/NEJMoa1800566.

14. "Labor Induction," Mayo Clinic, accessed July 9, 2019, https://www
    .mayoclinic.org/tests-procedures/labor-induction/about/pac-20385141.

15. Montse Palacio et al., "Meta-Analysis of Studies on Biochemical
    Marker Tests for the Diagnosis of Premature Rupture of Membranes:
    Comparison of Performance Indexes," BMC Pregnancy and Childbirth
    14, no. 183 (May 2014), https://doi.org/10.1186/1471-2393-14-183.

16. Labor and Maguire, "The Pain of Labour," https://doi.org/10.1177
    /204946370800200205.

17. H. G. Dahlen et al., "Perineal Outcomes and Maternal Comfort
    Related to the Application of Perineal Warm Packs in the Second Stage
    of Labor: A Randomized Controlled Trial," Birth 34, no. 4 (December
    2007): 282–90, https://doi.org/10.1111/j.1523-536X.2007.00186.x.

18. Shiliang Liu et al., "Maternal Mortality and Severe Morbidity Associated
    with Low-Risk Planned Cesarean Delivery Versus Planned Vaginal
    Delivery at Term," Canadian Medical Association Journal 176, no. 4
    (February 13, 2007): 455–60, https://doi.org/10.1503/cmaj.060870.

19. Guri Rortveit et al., "Urinary Incontinence After Vaginal Delivery or
    Cesarean Section," New England Journal of Medicine, no. 348 (March
    6, 2003): 900–907, https://doi.org/10.1056/NEJMoa021788.

20. H. E. Jakobsson et al., "Decreased Gut Microbiota Diversity, Delayed
    Bacteroidetes Colonisation and Reduced Th1 Responses in Infants
    Delivered by Caesarean Section," Gut 62, no. 4 (April 2014): 559–66,
    https://doi.org/10.1136/gutjnl-2012-303249.

21. "The Cost of Having a Baby in the United States," Truven
    Health Analytics, January 2013, http://www.chqpr.org/downloads/Cost
    ofHavingaBaby.pdf.

22. Andrea M. Carpentieri et al., "American Congress of Obstetricians and
    Gynecologists Survey on Professional Liability," American Congress
    of Obstetricians and Gynecologists, November 3, 2015, https://www
    .acog.org/-/media/Departments/Professional-Liability/2015PLSurvey
    NationalSummary11315.pdf?dmc=1&ts=20190401T192413242.

23. Mary E. Hannah, "Planned Elective Cesarean Section: A Reasonable
    Choice for Some Women?" Canadian Medical Association Journal 170,
    no. 5 (March 2, 2004): 813–14, https://doi.org/10.1503/cmaj.1032002.

24. "Delayed Umbilical Cord Clamping After Birth," American Col-
    lege of Obstetricians and Gynecologists, January 2017, https://
    www.acog.org/Clinical-Guidance-and-Publications/Committee
    -Opinions/Committee-on-Obstetric-Practice/Delayed-Umbilical
    -Cord-Clamping-After-Birth.

25. "Newborn Hearing Screening FAQs," American Academy of Pediatrics,

accessed July 2019, https://www.healthychildren.org/English/ages
-stages/baby/Pages/Purpose-of-Newborn-Hearing-Screening.aspx.

26. "Critical Congenital Heart Defects," Centers for Disease Control and
Prevention, accessed July 9, 2019, https://www.cdc.gov/ncbddd/heart
defects/cchd-facts.html.

# THE FOURTH TRIMESTER

1. A. R. Deussen, P. Ashwood, and R. Martis, "Analgesia for Relief of
Pains Due to Uterine Cramping/Involution After Birth," *Cochrane
Database of Systematic Reviews*, no. 5 (May 11, 2011), CD004908,
https://doi.org/10.1002/14651858.CD004908.pub2.

2. A. P. O'Brien et al., "New Fathers' Perinatal Depression and Anxiety-
Treatment Options: An Integrative Review," *American Journal of
Men's Health* 11, no. 4 (July 2017): 863–76, https://doi.org/10.1177
/1557988316669047.

## *Recovery*

1. "Maternity Care in the Netherlands," Naviva Kraamzorg, accessed
August 6, 2019, https://www.naviva.nl/naviva-kraamzorg-eng/.

2. "ACOG Redesigns Postpartum Care," American College of Obstetricians and Gynecologists, accessed August 8, 2019, https://www.acog
.org/About-ACOG/News-Room/News-Releases/2018/ACOG
-Redesigns-Postpartum-Care.

3. Jessica Keeler et al., "Diastasis Recti Abdominis: A Survey of Women's
Health Specialists for Current Physical Therapy Clinical Practice for
Postpartum Women," *Journal of Women's Health Physical Therapy* 36,
no. 3 (September/December 2012): 131–42, doi:10.1097/JWH.0b013
e318276f35f.

4. Oren S. Cheifetz et al., "The Effect of Abdominal Support on
Functional Outcomes in Patients Following Major Abdominal
Surgery: A Randomized Controlled Trial," *Physiotherapy Canada* 62,
no. 3 (2010): 242–53, accessed August 8, 2019, https://doi.org/10.3138
/physio.62.3.242.

5. Andrea Mary Woolner et al., "The Impact of Third- or Fourth-Degree
Perineal Tears on the Second Pregnancy: A Cohort Study of 182,445
Scottish Women," *PLoS ONE*, accessed August 8, 2019, https://doi
.org/10.1371/journal.pone.0215180.

6.   "Pelvic Organ Prolapse," A Fact Sheet from the Office on Women's Health, last accessed August 6, 2019, https://www.womenshealth.gov /files/documents/fact-sheet-pelvic-organ-prolapse.pdf.

7.   Abigail H. Garbarino et al., "Current Trends in Psychiatric Education Among Obstetrics and Gynecology Residency Programs," *Academic Psychiatry* 43, no. 3 (June 2019): 294–99, https://doi.org/10.1007/s405 96-019-01018-w.

8.   Elizabeth O'Connor et al., "Interventions to Prevent Perinatal Depression: Evidence Report and Systematic Review for the US Preventive Services Task Force," *JAMA* 321, no. 6 (2019): 588–601, doi:10.1001/jama.2018.20865.

### Your New Roommate

1.   Kate Wong, "Why Humans Give Birth to Helpless Babies," *Scientific American* (blog), August 28, 2012, accessed August 6, 2019, https:// blogs.scientificamerican.com/observations/why-humans-give-birth -to-helpless-babies/.

2.   "Who Breastfeeds in the United States?" Institute of Medicine (US) Committee on Nutritional Status During Pregnancy and Lactation, Washington (DC): National Academies Press (US); 1991, https://www .ncbi.nlm.nih.gov/books/NBK235588/.

3.   Mike Muller, "The Baby Killer," War on Want, March 1974, last accessed August 6, 2019. http://archive.babymilkaction.org/pdfs/babykiller.pdf.

4.   Jesse K. Anttila-Hughes et al., "Mortality from Nestlé's Marketing of Infant Formula in Low and Middle-Income Countries," National Bureau of Economic Research, March 2018, accessed August 8, 2019, https://www.nber.org/papers/w24452.

5.   "Infant Formula Market: Toddlers Milk Formula to Significantly Contribute to the Growth of the Overall Market: Global Industry Analysis (2012–2016) and Opportunity Assessment (2017–2027)," Future Market Insights, accessed August 8, 2019, https://www.future marketinsights.com/reports/infant-formula-market.

6.   "Breastfeeding Accessories Market Size, Share & Trends Analysis Report by Product (Nipple Care Products, Breast Shells, Breast Pads, Breastmilk Storage & Feeding), by Region, and Segment Forecasts, 2019–2026," Grand View Research, February 2019, accessed August 8, 2019, https://www.grandviewresearch.com/industry-analysis/breastfeeding -accessories-market.

7. "Breastfeeding and the Use of Human Milk," *Pediatrics* 129, no. 3 (March 2012), accessed August 8, 2019, https://pediatrics.aappublications.org/content/129/3/e827.

8. A. K. Ventura, "Does Breastfeeding Shape Food Preferences Links to Obesity," *Annals of Nutrition & Metabolism* 70, no. 3 (2017): 8–15, https://doi.org/10.1159/000478757.

9. "Breastfeeding Is an Investment in Health, Not Just a Lifestyle Decision," Centers for Disease Control and Prevention, accessed August 6, 2019, https://www.cdc.gov/breastfeeding/about-breastfeeding/why-it-matters.html.

10. Valerie Flaherman et al., "Health Care Utilization in the First Month After Birth and Its Relationship to Newborn Weight Loss and Method of Feeding," *Academic Pediatrics* 18, no. 6 (August 2018): 677–84, https://doi.org/10.1016/j.acap.2017.11.005.

11. "Breastfeeding Report Card," Centers for Disease Control and Prevention, accessed August 8, 2019, https://www.cdc.gov/breastfeeding/data/reportcard.htm.

12. "Employee Benefits Survey," US Bureau of Labor Statistics, accessed August 8, 2019, https://www.bls.gov/ncs/ebs/benefits/2014/ownership/civilian/table32a.htm.

13. Cynthia Reeves Tuttle and Wendy I. Slavitt, "Establishing the Business Case for Breastfeeding," *Breastfeeding Medicine* 4, no. s1 (October 14, 2009), https://doi.org/10.1089/bfm.2009.0031.

14. "The Physiological Basis of Breastfeeding," *Infant and Young Child Feeding: Model Chapter for Textbooks for Medical Students and Allied Health Professionals*, World Health Organization, 2009, https://www.ncbi.nlm.nih.gov/books/NBK148970/.

15. M. Papastavrou et al., "Breastfeeding in the Course of History," *Journal of Pediatrics and Neonatal Care* 2, no. 6 (September 2015), 00096, doi:10.15406/jpnc.2015.02.00096.

16. Emily E. Stevens, Thelma E. Patrick, and Rita Pickler, "A History of Infant Feeding," *Journal of Perinatal Education* 18, no. 2 (Spring 2009): 32–39, doi:10.1624/105812409X426314.

17. Anna Petherick, "Holder Pasteurization Has Limited Impact on the Nutrients in Human Milk," *Splash! Milk Science Update*, August 2017, https://milkgenomics.org/article/holder-pasteurization-limited-impact-nutrients-human-milk/.

18. Sarah A. Keim et al., "Cow's Milk Contamination of Human Milk Purchased Via the Internet," *Pediatrics* 135, no. 5 (May 2015): e1157–62, https://doi.org/10.1542/peds.2014-3554.

19. Carol L. Wilkinson et al., "Quantitative Evaluation of Content and Age Concordance Across Developmental Milestone Checklists," *Journal of Developmental and Behavioral Pediatrics*, June 4, 2019, https://doi .org/10.1097/DBP.0000000000000695.

## *Transitions*

1. Jennifer Barrett et al., "Maternal Affect and Quality of Parenting Experiences Are Related to Amygdala Response to Infant Faces," *Social Neuroscience* 7, no. 3 (2012): 252–68, https://doi.org/10.1080/1 7470919.2011.609907.
2. "Microchimerism," Wikipedia, accessed August 6, 2019, https:// en.wikipedia.org/wiki/Microchimerism.
3. O. Lapaire et al., "Georg Schmorl on Trophoblasts in the Maternal Circulation," *Placenta* 28, no. 1 (January 2007): 1–5, https://doi .org/10.1016/j.placenta.2006.02.004.
4. Amy M. Boddy et al., "Fetal Microchimerism and Maternal Health: A Review and Evolutionary Analysis of Cooperation and Conflict Beyond the Womb," *BioEssays* 37, no. 10 (October 2015): 1106–18, https://doi.org/10.1002/bies.201500059.
5. K. A. Guthrie et al., "Parity and HLA alleles in risk of rheumatoid arthritis," *Chimerism* 2, no. 1 (January 2011): 11–15, doi:10.4161/chim .2.1.15424.
6. Michael Verneris, "Fetal Microchimerism—What Our Children Leave Behind," *Blood* 102, no. 10 (2003): 3465–66, https://doi.org/10.1182 /blood-2003-09-3027.

# INDEX

**Note:** Page references in italics indicate illustrations, and a *t* indicates a table.